WHAT TEST-TAKERS ARE SAYING ABOUT LEARNINGEXPRESS PREPARATION GUIDES

"The information from the last two study guides I ordered from your company was invaluable.... Better than the $200 6-week study courses being offered.... After studying from dozens of books I would choose yours over any of the other companies."
S. Frosch

"Excellent . . . It was like having the test in advance!"
J. Kennedy

"Without this book, I wouldn't have understood the test."
R. Diaz

"Told me everything that was going to be on the test [and] gave me a good understanding of the whole process, too."
J. Molinari

"The best test-prep book I've used!"
H. Hernandez

SANITATION WORKER EXAM

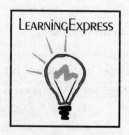

LEARNINGEXPRESS

NEW YORK

Copyright © 1997 Learning Express, LLC.

All rights reserved under International and Pan-American Copyright Conventions. Published in the United States by LearningExpress, LLC, New York.

Library of Congress Cataloging-in-Publication Data

Sanitation worker exam: national edition. — 1st ed.
    p.   cm. — (LearningExpress civil service library)
  ISBN 1-57685-047-1
  1. Sanitation workers—Examinations,
questions, etc.   2. Refuse collection—Vocational guidance
I. Series.
TD794.S25   1997
363.72'009747'1—DC21

97-22390
CIP

Printed in the United States of America
9 8 7 6 5 4 3 2 1
First Edition

Regarding the Information in this Book
We attempt to verify the information presented in our books prior to publication. It is always a good idea, however, to double-check such important information as minimum requirements, application and testing procedures, and deadlines with your local hiring agency, as such information can change from time to time.

For Further Information
For information on LearningExpress, other LearningExpress products, or bulk sales, please call or write to us at:
    LearningExpress®
    900 Broadway
    Suite 604
    New York, NY 10003
    212-995-2566

LearningExpress is an affiliated company of Random House, Inc.

Distributed to the retail trade by Random House, Inc., as agent for LearningExpress, LLC.
Visit LearningExpress on the World Wide Web at www.learnx.com.

ISBN 1-57685-047-1

7 85555 85047 7

CONTENTS

LIST OF CONTRIBUTORS

The following individuals contributed to the content of this book.

Elizabeth Chesla is an adult educator and curriculum developer at Polytechnic University in New York who has also taught reading and writing at New York University School of Continuing Education and New York Institute of Technology in New York City.

Jan Gallagher, Ph.D., is a test-development specialist, editor, and teacher living in Jersey City, New Jersey.

Mary Hesalroad, a former police officer for the Austin, Texas, Police Department, consults with police departments on recruiting efforts and is a freelance writer now living in San Marcos, Texas.

Judith N. Meyers is an instructor in reading and study skills at Wagner College, Staten Island, New York; director of the Two Together Tutorial Program of the Jewish Child Care Association in New York City; and an Adult Basic Education Practitioner at City University New York.

Judith F. Olson, M.A., is chairperson of the language arts department at Valley High School in West Des Moines, Iowa, where she also conducts test preparation workshops.

Judith Robinovitz is an independent educational consultant and director of Score At the Top, a comprehensive test preparation program in Vero Beach, Florida.

Jo Lynn Southard is a freelance writer and editor living in Portland, Maine.

The following LearningExpress staff members also contributed to the writing and researching of this book: **Jean Eckhoff** and **Edward Grossman**.

C·H·A·P·T·E·R 1

HOW TO BECOME A SANITATION WORKER

CHAPTER SUMMARY

If you're interested in becoming a sanitation worker, this chapter will give you information on the application process, the tests you may be required to take, and any special licenses you may need to have. While sanitation operations vary from place to place, this chapter outlines hiring procedures that are commonly found in sanitation departments.

Sanitation workers (who may also be called refuse collectors) are vital to the smooth—and clean!—operation of any city or town. Sanitation departments traditionally are responsible for picking up residential trash and cleaning streets. In the last few years, however, these departments have also become concerned with recycling and with hazardous waste disposal.

The main job of a sanitation worker is to drive or ride a sanitation truck, stopping frequently to pick up trash that residents have placed on the curb. In addition, sanitation workers now pick up and sort recyclables, dispose of hazardous waste, clean streets and alleys, and even help out with snow removal! If you enjoy working outside, in a job where you get to work without a great deal of supervision and do a variety of different tasks, sanitation work may be for you.

Sanitation workers, not surprisingly, must be able to do strenuous physical labor, including lifting and carrying heavy trash cans. A sanitation worker will most often work the first shift, so if you are a "morning person" or like the idea of having your late afternoons free, sanitation may be a good job for you. In northern cities, sanitation workers may also run snow plows, either every time streets need to be cleaned or as additional plow operators when snows are particularly heavy. For this reason, you may be required to live within the city where you work, in order to get to work quickly in a snow emergency.

Being a sanitation worker may not be the most glamorous job in the world, but without question, it's an important one. If you've ever been in a city during a garbage strike, you know how necessary sanitation workers are. Or, look out on your street the next garbage day before the trucks come to haul away the trash. Imagine what your street would look like if the trucks didn't come this week . . . or next week . . . or the week after that. Then imagine that no one empties the trash cans downtown on the street corners or in the park. And the streets are never cleaned or cleared of snow. Sanitation workers do all these things—and more—that make our lives easier and more pleasant.

Sanitation Workers Strike It Rich!

In less than a month, 29 different sanitation workers in Louisville, Kentucky, won three different lottery games, for a total of $17.4 million! First, a group of 17 workers at a waste management company won $15 million in Lotto Kentucky. Three weeks later, a group of 11 workers at an industrial disposal company, who never pooled their money until they heard of the other group's luck, won $2.3 million in Lotto Kentucky. Four days after that, a sanitation worker for the City of Louisville won $100,000 in the Kentucky Lottery's Cash 5 game. Nice work if you can get it!

So if you think you would like being out-of-doors, working independently, and performing services that are vital to your community, look into being a sanitation worker. The need for sanitation workers can only increase in the future, as the population increases and as we expect our cities to provide a greater variety of solid waste services, like recycling and hazardous waste disposal. That means that sanitation worker jobs will become more competitive over the next few years, as cities take on more sanitation responsibilities. This book will prepare you to be successful in applying for and winning a sanitation worker position.

APPLYING TO BECOME A SANITATION WORKER

MINIMUM REQUIREMENTS

Sanitation work varies from community to community. In some cases, it is performed by private companies that contract with the city; most often, though, the city or county government provides sanitation services. After all, it's one of the things we pay taxes for! Because the work varies, so do the minimum requirements for the job. Almost everywhere, though, you will need to be at least 18 years old. In almost every case, too, you will need to demonstrate that you can understand and follow directions and communicate effectively. And no matter where you perform the job of sanitation worker, you will need physical strength, agility, and stamina.

In many cases, you will also need a Commercial Driver's License (CDL) in order to be a sanitation worker. A crew of sanitation workers is usually made up of two or three people—one to drive the truck and one or two to empty the cans and operate the compaction equipment. Sometimes, the members of these crews rotate among jobs and then all of them need to have a CDL—usually a Class A or Class B, with air brakes certification. In some areas, however, truck drivers and garbage collectors are separate jobs with different hiring standards and you would not need a CDL to be a garbage collector. Even then, however, you will probably want to get a CDL eventually, as becoming a truck driver usually means a promotion—and a raise in pay!

As noted above, you may be required, after you are hired, to live within the city limits or within a certain distance from the sanitation facility, so you can get to work in a hurry in case of an emergency. And that's about it as far as minimum requirements go. In most cases, there are not formal education requirements (that is, you don't have to have a High School diploma or GED). Usually, too, there are no formal requirements as to the job experience you must have. What you need most are a strong back, the ability to work without supervision, and a desire to work outside, performing a public service.

It is important to note once again that there is a great deal of variety among sanitation jobs. It is vital that you check the requirements for the city you are interested in before you apply. If the department is advertising for employees, the job announcement will contain all the information you need to know about the city's minimum requirements. If they take applications all the time and keep them on file for an opening, the personnel department can tell you what the minimum requirements are.

SELECTION PROCESS

A typical selection process for becoming a sanitation worker includes some or all of the following steps:

1. Fill out an application
2. Take a written examination
3. Take an agility and strength test or a performance evaluation
4. Be interviewed by your potential boss

5. Have a physical—usually performed by a doctor that the city chooses
6. Submit to a drug and alcohol screening

The Application

The first thing you need to do is find out where to get an application. A good place to start is your city's Personnel office. This office may also be called Human Resources. They can usually tell you, first, if they are in charge of the applications for this particular job and, second, if applications are currently being accepted.

In some cities, sanitation worker applications are accepted at any time; after an applicant has completed the application and, possibly, the interview, they are usually added to the eligibility list along with other applicants. (The city usually doesn't want to pay for your physical and drug screen until they have made you a conditional offer of employment—that is, an offer for a job that is conditioned on your passing the physical and drug screen.) In other cities, applications are accepted only when the Department of Sanitation actually has openings. The personnel office can tell you where to watch for announcements of these openings.

One thing that can be very confusing in the job application process is simply finding the right department to give you information. In some cases, instead of the city Personnel office, the Department of Sanitation does its own hiring. Only it may not be called the Department of Sanitation. It may be the Bureau of Solid Waste, or the Streets and Sanitation Division, or the Refuse Collection Department. You may just have to ask, "What department is in charge of picking up trash?"

After you find out who distributes and collects the applications and when they are being accepted, you will need to fill out the application. In most cases, this will be a standard employment application that asks about your educational history and employment experience.

Make sure you fill out the application completely and neatly, being careful to follow all directions accurately.

Often, when applying for government jobs, you will need to submit copies of other documents along with your application. Usually, this will include some sort of proof that you may legally be hired in the U.S., such as a birth certificate or citizenship certificate, or proof that you are a legal alien if you are not a citizen. In cases where you need to have or obtain a CDL, you may need to turn in a copy of that and a copy of your driving record. If you served in the military, you may need to provide copies of your discharge papers. Although it is unusual, if you apply in a city that requires you to have a High School diploma or GED, you will need to supply a copy of that. Whatever you need to hand in with your application will be listed on the application itself or on the job announcement. Make sure you turn in your application only when it is complete.

Chapter 3 offers further practical advice on filling out a civil service application and includes a sample application.

The Written Examination

If you are required to take a written examination, it will likely be one of two basic kinds. It may test your reading comprehension, your ability to follow directions, and your skill at reading maps and schedules; or it may test your knowledge of safe driving practices and the operation of various kinds if trucks. A third alternative is that the exam may test all of these areas. Later chapters of this book address various techniques you can use to prepare for these tests and offer three complete practice exams so you can sharpen your test-taking skills.

Usually, the job announcement will give you information about the skills the exam is designed to test. If not, someone in the Personnel department can tell you. For an entry-level job, you usually will not be expected to know about specific laws and regulations that relate to sanitation in your city. Obviously, if the job you are applying for does not require you to have a CDL, because you are not going to be driving a truck, you won't be tested on driving safety or truck operation.

The Agility and Strength Test

Some sanitation departments require you to demonstrate your physical ability to do the job by passing an agility and strength test. Many others do not. Chapter 13, "The Physical Test," describes a typical test and shows you how to prepare for this hurdle in the hiring process. Whether you have to take this test or not, you'll still want to see if you can do these exercises!

The Performance Test

In some cities, you may also be required to take a performance test in order to be hired for a sanitation position. Just what skills are tested depends on the description of the job you are applying for.

If the position you are interested in includes driving a refuse collection truck, you may be required to demonstrate that you know how to operate the truck safely. This performance test will be very similar to the driving test the state gives when issuing a CDL. If you are required to have a CDL in order to apply for the job, chances are you are already quite familiar with safe operation of a truck. The test will either take place in a secured area, such as an empty parking lot, or, as long as you have a CDL or permit, out on the street in traffic. It may be a combination of both.

Sanitation truck drivers are required to perform maneuvers that can get in the way of other traffic. You need to demonstrate that you can perform these actions as safely and efficiently as possible. For example, sanitation trucks must pull over near the curb in order to allow the truck to be loaded with garbage. You should be able to do this in a way that keeps the truck as far as possible out of the flow of traffic while at the same time making sure you don't get caught, behind a parked car for example, so that you can't drive the truck on to the next stop. Sometimes sanitation trucks have to pull over on the "wrong" side of the road; you need to be able to do this as safely as possible. In addition, when driving in traffic, you need to demonstrate to your potential boss that you are familiar with the rules of the road and that you follow them.

A Note About CDLs

Not all sanitation worker positions require you to have a Commercial Driver's License in order to apply for the job. If the job you are interested in requires you to drive a sanitation truck, at least part of the time, you will obviously need a CDL. However, even if you are not required to have a CDL in order to be hired for the job, you may want to get one soon after you get hired, since that may be the fastest way to promotion and higher pay. Find out if the Sanitation Department will help you prepare for the CDL exam. Also, federal law requires that you pass a physical in order to receive a CDL; check with your state Department of Motor Vehicles or Transportation.

The other kind of performance evaluation you may be required to take is one that tests your strength, stamina, and flexibility. Usually, the job description for sanitation workers states that you must be able to lift and carry 50 pounds. In some areas, it may be up to 75 pounds. One goal of the performance evaluation is to assure than you can lift and carry the necessary amount. If you can't, you won't be able to do the job. The evaluation is essentially the same as the agility and strength test that is discussed in Chapter 13, only you are not competing with other candidates; your bosses use it as a way of making sure you can handle the job and to see in what areas you might need some extra training. See Chapter 13 for some ideas on how to prepare for this evaluation.

Of course, depending on the details of the job description of the position you are applying for, you may have to go through both of these performance evaluations.

The Interview

One of the biggest mistakes people make in applying for a job is in not preparing for the interview. We all seem to think that there's nothing we can do to get ready. But a little thought and maybe even some discussion with a friend or partner can do a great deal toward preparing you for the dreaded job interview.

Start by thinking about the information on your job application. (You may even want to keep a copy of it—especially if it is going to be a while before your interview.) There are some things on your application that you can almost guarantee you'll be asked about. For example, if there is a large gap in your work history, be prepared to talk about it. Be ready to talk about why you quit or were fired from a previous job. These are not necessarily bad things, and if you are prepared, you can talk about them in the best light. For example, it is probably not a good idea to say you quit an earlier job because you were bored, but you can say that, while the job was initially challenging, after a while you realized there seemed to be no possibility of advancement.

Always be honest in a job interview. Chances are that when you signed your job application, you gave the Sanitation Department permission to verify information you gave them. Don't say you quit a job when you were fired, or lie about the dates you worked somewhere to cover up a period of unemployment. Almost everyone has been fired at least once and has spent some time unemployed. Just tell the truth and present your situation in the best light.

The Medical Exam and Drug and Alcohol Screen

Because sanitation workers need to be strong, agile, and generally healthy, chances are you will be required to have a physical exam performed by a doctor before you can be hired by a sanitation department. Usually, this will only happen after you are offered conditional employment—that is, conditional on passing the physical. The sanitation department will pay for the exam and, most often, it will be done by a doctor or clinic that they choose.

Most likely you have had a physical before. You know that there is some variety in the way doctors perform physicals, but, generally, the doctor will check your heart, lungs, reflexes, vision, blood pressure, temperature, and so forth. In addition, this physical will check some things specific to the sanitation worker job. Doctors call this a "functional capacity evaluation" or a "human performance evaluation." All that means is that they want to make sure you can do all the things required in this job.

The doctor will want to test your strength (for lifting and carrying), your stamina (for long hours of physical work), and your flexibility (for picking up and setting down garbage cans and bags). Different doctors will do this in different ways. They may have you lift a weight or use a resistance machine, have you take a treadmill test or other workout, or have you perform a series of bends and stretches. The point of any of the tests they do is to simulate the requirements of the job. See Chapter 13 on the agility and strength test for an idea of the kinds of things you might be expected to do.

There's really not much you can do to prepare for the physical exam. As you can see by the kinds of things you may have to do for the functional capacity evaluation, it would be a good idea to be well rested for the exam. Also, wear comfortable, loose-fitting clothes and do some stretches to limber up before you start.

In most cases, you will be required to undergo a drug and alcohol screen prior to employment and random checks while you are employed.

ON THE JOB

After you make it through the hiring process and the physicals, you can begin your job as a sanitation worker. Usually, you will be trained "on the job" by senior employees. In some cases, there will be a few hours of classroom work, followed by some hands-on training at a sanitation facility before you go out on the street. You won't be expected to work on your own until you are familiar with all the equipment and procedures; even then, sanitation workers usually work in teams of two or three.

A One-Man Show

New hydraulic load and pack vehicles enable sanitation workers to work individually, rather than in teams of one truck driver and one or two refuse collectors. Currently only in very limited use, these vehicles have hydraulic arms that pick up trash cans and empty them into containers on the back of the truck. This container then compacts the trash while the driver continues on to the next pick up spot. An experienced operator can direct the arm to grasp the can, pick it up, empty it into the container, and return it to the ground in five seconds!

WORK HOURS

Once you are through with training and are a regular sanitation worker, you will most likely be assigned to regular routes on specific days. Chances are, you will work "first shift," that is, 6:00 or 7:00 a.m. to 2:00 or 3:00 p.m. This schedule is one of the things many people feel is an advantage to sanitation work. Certainly, if you are a morning person, there is still a lot of the day left after work for you to do other things.

Another possibility is the third shift, say from 11:00 p.m. to 7:00 a.m. In most cases, workers on this shift empty trash cans downtown, in parks, and other public areas. Again, many people enjoy working the third shift and you might want to try it and see if it works for you. The least common shift assignment for sanitation workers is the second shift, afternoon and evening. In some cities, sanitation workers will empty dumpsters at schools and other public buildings on second shift, but usually this is done by workers on other shifts.

SALARY, RAISES, AND PROMOTIONS

Most sanitation workforces are unionized. Among the unions representing sanitation workers are the Teamsters and the American Federation of State, County, and Municipal Employees. Laws vary from state to state on whether your workforce is a "union shop"—that is, everyone on the job must join the union—or a "right to work" shop—where you can choose to join the union or not. The union presence among sanitation workers has improved the job tremendously over the last few decades. Sanitation workers are generally well-paid and enjoy job security. They receive, thanks to the unions, regular raises and promotions. The unions have taken us from the days of "garbage men" to today, the era of sanitation workers.

United We Stand
The International Brotherhood of Teamsters headquarters is located at:
25 Louisiana Ave., N.W.
Washington, D.C. 20001
202-624-6800
http://www.teamsters.org
The American Federation of State, County, and Municipal Employees (AFSCME) headquarters is located at:
1625 L St. N.W.
Washington, D.C. 20036
202-429-1130
http://www.afscme.org

The following table presents the starting salaries for sanitation workers in six major cities, to give you an idea of the kind of starting wage you can expect.

In some cases, sanitation workers may receive a night shift differential if they work the third shift, making their staring wage even higher. Because sanitation workers are usually city employees, as well as union members, benefits such as vacations, sick leave, insurance, and retirement are usually comparatively good. For the same reasons, the jobs are usually secure.

Promotional opportunities vary among sanitation departments. In many cases, however, Sanitation Truck Operator is the first promotion you might

SALARY: AT A GLANCE

Position	Monthly Salary	Annual Salary
Chicago, Illinois	$3,285.00	$39,416.00
Detroit, Michigan	$1,613.73	$19,364.80
Indianapolis, Indiana	$2,019.34	$24,232.00
New York City	$2,063.00	$24,758.00
Portland, Maine	$1,958.67	$23,504.00

become eligible for. Obviously, you will have to have a CDL for this job, so many people like to get their CDL shortly after they are hired in a sanitation department, to increase their chances for promotion. Either formally or informally, senior employees can help you prepare for your CDL; in some cities, the sanitation department will pay some or all of the cost of obtaining your license. Be sure to check with your supervisor before you proceed with getting your CDL.

THE FUTURE

Sanitation workers are vital to the smooth functioning of any city. It is a job that provides the opportunity to work independently and plenty of variety. Sanitation workers not only pick up trash in residential areas, they pick up and sort recyclables, empty dumpsters at public buildings and baskets in public parks, clean streets, and even, on occasion, dispose of hazardous materials.

Over the last several decades, we've become aware that we can't just continue to haul things to the landfill; we're running out of room. So more and more cities are instituting recycling programs and hazardous waste disposal programs, in hopes of finding more efficient ways of dealing with all the waste we create. As long as these programs continue to grow, sanitation workers will always be in demand. What could be better than an important job, that is also well-paying and secure?

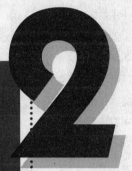

C·H·A·P·T·E·R 2

HIRING PROCEDURES FOR MAJOR U.S. CITIES

CHAPTER SUMMARY

This chapter presents a goldmine of information: minimum requirements and hiring procedures for sanitation workers at top cities around the country. Use the information presented in these profiles to get the specific information you need to apply for a job in these cities—or just generally to find out what's likely to be required of you to get a sanitation job in your city.

One of the keys to becoming a sanitation worker is knowing what the minimum requirements are and how the hiring process works. Just keeping on top of those basics will help you stand out from the crowd and win the job you want.

The following pages present a rundown of important information on how sanitation workers are hired in 26 major cities in the U.S. Even if your city isn't among those listed, chances are its hiring procedures will be similar to those listed here. Be sure to contact the personnel department of your local agency for all the particulars, though.

For most cities, a job information hot line is included to help you stay on top of all the possible opportunities in your area. The cities listed here are presented in alphabetical order.

AUSTIN, TEXAS

Hiring Agency

Department of Personnel
206 E 9th Street, 1st Floor
Austin, TX 78701
Phone: 512-499-3272
Job Info/Test Line: 1-800-526-9159

Minimum Requirements

Age: 18
Education: None
Driver's License/Record: None
Other: 6 months related experience: construction or labor

Hiring Procedures

1. Application
2. Interview
3. Reference Check
4. Drug Test

BALTIMORE, MARYLAND

Hiring Agency

Department of Personnel Classification Dept.
201 East Baltimore Street
Phone: 410-396-3877
Job Info/Test Line: 410-396-3860

Minimum Requirements

Age: None
Education: None
Driver's License/Record: None
Citizenship: Preferred but not required
Other: Ability to lift heavy objects, bend and stretch. Ability to read, write and follow directions.

Hiring Procedures

1. Application
2. Interview

BOSTON, MASSACHUSETTS

Hiring Agency

Waste Management
204 Merrimac Street
Woburn, MA 01801
Phone: 617-933-2113
Job Info/Test Line: 1-888-222-6648

Minimum Requirements

Age: 18; 21 for drivers
Education: None
Driver's License/Record: CDL
Citizenship: None
Other: Ability to perform strenuous physical exertion in all seasons outdoors.

Hiring Procedures

1. Telephone Application
2. Interview
3. Background Check
4. Drug Screen
5. Physical Evaluation

CHICAGO, ILLINOIS

Hiring Agency

City Dept. of Personnel (Service Center)
121 North LaSalle, Room 100
Chicago, IL 60602
Phone: 312-744-4976
Job Info/Test Line: 312-744-1369

Minimum Requirements

Age: None
Education: None

Driver's License/Record: No specific license required
Citizenship: None
Other: Good Physical Condition and ability to read and write

Hiring Procedures

1. Application-put in a lottery
2. Questionnaire (Interview)
3. Physical (Medical)
4. Orientation

CLEVELAND, OHIO

Hiring Agency

City Department of Personnel
601 Lakeside Avenue
Cleveland, OH 44114
Phone: 216-664-2000
Job Info/Test Line: 216-664-2420

Minimum Requirements

Age: None
Education: Completion of 8th Grade
Driver's License/Record: None
Citizenship: U.S. Citizenship and Residency required
Other: Ability to lift 50 lbs.

Hiring Procedures

1. Application
2. Interview
3. Physical
4. Drug Screen

COLUMBUS, OHIO

Hiring Agency

Civil Service Commission
50 West Gay Street, Room 600

Columbus, OH 43215
Phone: 614-645-8300
Job Info/Test Line: 614-645-7667

Minimum Requirements

Age: None
Education: None
Driver's License/Record: CDL
Citizenship: US Citizen; Resident of Franklin County or any of the surrounding counties
Other: One year experience in sanitation or operating a truck

Hiring Procedures

1. Application
2. Performance Exam
3. Interview

DALLAS, TEXAS

Hiring Agency

City Department of Human Resources
1500 Marilla Street, Room 6A North
Dallas, TX 75201
Phone: 214-670-3710
Job Info/Test Line: 214-670-5908

Minimum Requirements

Age: None
Education: None
Driver's License/Record: CDL
Citizenship: None
Other: Ability to perform manual labor for an extended period of time; ability to lift 50 lbs; ability to use a variety of tools.

Hiring Procedures

1. Application
2. Drug Screen

DETROIT, MICHIGAN

Hiring Agency

City Department of Human Resources

2 Woodward Avenue

Detroit, MI 48226

Phone: 313-224-3714

Job Info/Test Line: 313-224-6928

Minimum Requirements

Age: None

Education: High School Diploma preferred but not required

Driver's License/Record: CDL Class A or B

Citizenship: Residency required upon hire

Hiring Procedures

1. Application
2. Written Exam
3. Drug Screen
4. Medical

EL PASO, TEXAS

Hiring Agency

City Department of Personnel

2 Civic Center Plaza

El Paso, TX 79901

Phone: 915-541-4505

Job Info/Test Line: 915-541-4094

Minimum Requirements

Age: None

Education: None

Driver's License/Record: None (CDL Class B for Driver Position)

Citizenship: U.S. Citizenship

Hiring Procedures

1. Application
2. Written Examination
3. Interview
4. Drug Screen

HOUSTON, TEXAS

Hiring Agency

City Department of Personnel

500 Jefferson Street, 15th Floor

Phone: 713-658-3717

Job Info/Test Line: 713-658-3798

Minimum Requirements

Age: 18

Education: Completion of 8th grade

Citizenship: U.S. Citizenship

Other: Ability to lift 80 lbs.

Hiring Procedures

1. Application
2. Interview
3. Drug Screen

INDIANAPOLIS, INDIANA

Hiring Agency

City of Indianapolis HR Department

200 East Washington, Room 1501

Indianapolis, IN 46204

Phone: 317-327-5200

Job Info/Test Line: 317-327-5191

Minimum Requirements

Age: 18

Education: None

Driver's License/Record: None

Citizenship: None

Other: Good physical condition

Hiring Procedures

1. Application and Fingerprinting
   (for background investigation)
2. Interview
3. Orientation

JACKSONVILLE, FLORIDA

Hiring Agency

City Personnel Department
220 East Bay Street, Room 113
Jacksonville, FL 32202
Phone: 904-630-1111
Job Info/Test Line: 904-630-1144

Minimum Requirements

Age: None
Education: None
Driver's License/Record: Preferred, but
     not required
Citizenship: None to apply;
     eventual U.S. Citizenship required

Hiring Procedures

1. Application
2. Drug screening
3. Interview
4. Background Investigation

LOS ANGELES, CALIFORNIA

Hiring Agency

Department of Personnel
Recruitment Division, Room 100
700 East Temple Street
Los Angeles, CA 90012
Phone: 213-847-9241
Job Info/Test Line: 213-847-9424

Minimum Requirements

Age: None
Education: None
Driver's License/Record: CDL Class B
Citizenship: U.S. Citizen or Resident
Other: One year experience as a Truck Operator

Hiring Procedures

1. Application
2. Written Examination
3. Performance Test

MEMPHIS, TENNESSEE

Hiring Agency

City Department of Personnel
125 North Lane
Memphis, TN 38103
Phone: 901-576-6509
Job Info/Test Line: 901-576-6548

Minimum Requirements

Age: 18
Education: None
Driver's License/Record: CDL Class B. (For driver
     position: the ability to operate a variety
     of trucks.)
Citizenship: Residency Requirement
Other: Ability to understand written and verbal
     instructions. Ability to bend, kneel, stretch
     and lift 50 lbs. unassisted.

Hiring Procedures

1. Application
2. Interview
3. Drug Screen
4. Background Investigation (Police Record)

MILWAUKEE, WISCONSIN

Hiring Agency

City of Milwaukee Department of Employee
Relations
200 East Wells Street
Milwaukee, WI 53202
Phone: 414-286-3751
Job Info/Test Line: 414-286-5555

Minimum Requirements

Age: 18
Education: None
Driver's License/Record: None
Citizenship: Resident of Milwaukee
Other: Good Physical Condition

Hiring Procedures

1. Application
2. Written Examination
3. Strength Agility
4. Eligible List
5. Interview
6. Physical (Medical)
7. Appointment

Notes

To be considered for the position of Sanitation
Laborer, an applicant must first be employed as
a City Laborer.

NASHVILLE, TENNESSEE

Hiring Agency

City Department of Personnel
222 3d Avenue North
Nashville, TN 37201
Phone: 615-862-6640
Job Info/Test Line: 615-862-6660

Minimum Requirements

Age: None
Education: Completion of 8th Grade
Driver's License/Record: None
Citizenship: U.S. Citizenship

Hiring Procedures

1. Application
2. Interview

NEW YORK, NY

Hiring Agency

Dept. of Citywide Administrative Services-
Application Section
18 Washington Street
New York, NY 10004
Phone: 212-487-6500 (includes Job/Test Info)

Minimum Requirements

Age: 18-21
Education: None
Driver's License/Record: CDL Class A or B
Citizenship: Resident of NYC, Nassau or
        Westchester County
Other: Ability to understand and be
        understood in English

Hiring Procedures

1. Application
2. Written Examination
3. Physical Test
4. Conditional offer of Employment
5. Medical Examination and Drug Test

PHILADELPHIA, PENNSYLVANIA

Hiring Agency

City Department of Personnel
1401 JFK Boulevard

Philadelphia, PA 19102
Phone: 215-686-2347

Minimum Requirements

Age: None
Education: None
Driver's License/Record: CDL
Citizenship: Resident of Philadelphia
Other: Ability to understand and carry out instructions

Hiring Procedures

1. Applications
2. Placed in a lottery
3. Physical Evaluation

PHOENIX, ARIZONA
Hiring Agency

City Personnel, Employment and Training Division
135 North 2nd Avenue
Phoenix, AZ 85003
Phone: 602-262-7562
Job Info/Test Line: 602-252-5627

Minimum Requirements

Age: 18
Education: None
Driver's License/Record: CDL Class A
Citizenship: Resident of Maricopa County
Other: Ability to lift 50 lbs.

Hiring Procedures

1. Application
2. Interview
3. Drug Screen
4. Medical Evaluation

SAN ANTONIO, TEXAS
Hiring Agency

City of San Antonio HR Dept.
111 Plaza DeArmes
San Antonio, TX 78205
Phone: 210-207-8108
Job Info/Test Line: 210-207-7280

Minimum Requirements

Age: 18
Education: None
Driver's License/Record: Possess a CDL License
Citizenship: U.S. Citizen or Resident
Other: Good physical condition and ability to read and write

Hiring Procedures

1. Application
2. Interview
3. Physical Evaluation
4. Orientation

Notes

After applications have been accepted by the HR Department, they are sent to the Solid Waste Division of Public Works, where they review the applications again and conduct the interviews. The applicants selected are sent back to the HR Department to go through a physical evaluation and orientation.

SAN DIEGO, CALIFORNIA
Hiring Agency

Department of Personnel
1200 3rd Avenue, Suite 101
Phone: 619-236-6400
Job Info/Test Line: 619-682-1011

Minimum Requirements

Age: 18
Education: None
Driver's License/Record: CDL Class B
Citizenship: None
Other: Ability to lift 65 lbs.

Hiring Procedures

1. Application
2. Interview

SAN FRANCISCO, CALIFORNIA

Hiring Agency

Golden Gate Disposal
Address: 900 7th Avenue
San Francisco, CA 94107
Phone: 415-626-4000

Minimum Requirements

Age: 21-40
Education: High School Diploma
Driver's License/Record: CDL Class B
Other: Ability to lift heavy objects using
knees and back

Hiring Procedures

1. Application
2. Interview
3. Drug Screen
4. Physical

Notes

Golden Gate Disposal is one of the two private contractors that handle garbage disposal in San Francisco. The other private contractor is Sunset Scavenger.

SAN JOSE, CALIFORNIA

Hiring Agency

Green Team
1333 Oakland Road
San Jose, CA 95112
Phone: 408-283-8500

Minimum Requirements

Age: None
Education: None
Driver's License/Record: CDL Class A or B
with Air Brakes
Citizenship: U.S.

Hiring Procedures

1. Application
2. Interview

Notes

Green Team is one of the two private contractors that handle garbage disposal in San Francisco. The other private contractor is Western Waste.

SEATTLE, WASHINGTON

Hiring Agency

US Disposal
500 South Sullivan Street
Seattle, WA 98108
Phone: 206-646-2526

Minimum Requirements

Age: None
Education: None
Driver's License/Record: CDL Class A or B
Citizenship: None

Hiring Procedures

1. Application
2. Interview
3. Drug Screen
4. Physical

Notes

US Disposal is a Private Contractor.

SEATTLE, WASHINGTON
Hiring Agency

General Disposal
14-15 NW Ballard Way
Seattle, WA 98107
Phone: 206-782-3535

Minimum Requirements

Age: 18
Education: None
Driver's License/Record: CDL Class B
Citizenship: None
Other: Ability to lift heavy objects

Hiring Procedures

Individuals interested in a position with General Disposal report to the "yard" and are picked for employment. They must possess a CDL Class B license. Seniority is given to those picked first, who then fill out an application.

Notes

General Disposal is a Private Contractor.

WASHINGTON, DC
Hiring Agency

DC Department of Personnel
2000 14th Street NW, Room 325
Washington, DC 20009
Phone: 202-939-8730

Minimum Requirements

Age: 18
Education: None
Driver's License/Record: CDL
Other: Ability to lift 50-70 lbs.

Hiring Procedures

1. Application
2. Interview

FILLING OUT A CIVIL SERVICE APPLICATION 3

CHAPTER SUMMARY

Filling out an application is usually the first step in applying for a job working for local government. It's your first (and maybe your last!) chance to make a good impression. This chapter shows you how to avoid common application mistakes while putting your best foot forward so that you come out a step ahead.

magine this. You work in the personnel department of a huge civil service agency. You've just been handed 100 applications and your boss asks you to check through them to make sure each applicant meets the minimum qualifications for the job. Oh. And there's 2,900 more where that came from, so when you're done . . . .

This situation was *not* make-believe for human resource specialists in a large civil service department in the state of Washington in 1996. They had to examine over 3,000 applications before the field was narrowed down to the 250 people they hired that year. It's overwhelming to even imagine reading that much material—almost as overwhelming as thinking about *your* application being one of 3,000 someone has to read. How on earth can you compete against all those people?

THE REAL ENEMY

Here's a secret . . . you aren't competing against anyone but yourself at this stage of the game. It might surprise you to hear that in the example mentioned above, over 50% of the applications submitted were rejected before the applicant reached the interview stage. They weren't rejected because another applicant beat them out, but because they didn't meet the minimum qualifications for applying in the first place *and/or* because their applications weren't properly completed.

According to personnel specialists from many of the major civil service agencies, all applications are screened first to see if the applicant meets minimum qualifications. For example, if the agency requires all applicants to have a high school diploma and you do not have one then your application will most likely see the reject pile. Save yourself a bit of disappointment by carefully checking the requirements for sanitation worker <u>before</u> you fill out the application. And don't be afraid to ask questions if you have doubts about whether you meet the requirements.

You might not have much control over whether or not you meet minimum requirements at the time you apply for sanitation worker, but you have 100% control over the first impression you make on your potential employer. That first impression will be made, in most cases, with the written application.

Let's face it, paperwork is tedious and most people believe that no one reads their applications or resumes anyway. This is the Sirens' call for the unsuccessful—don't listen! Not only will agencies and sanitation companies thoroughly scrutinize your written application for sanitation worker, this document will be judged and assigned a point value in many of the hiring systems in use nationwide. The written application is a fantastic opportunity for you to earn brownie points and build up a solid reputation with your potential employer.

Here are some tips from the biggest sanitation worker employers across the nation for turning in a winning application.

READ THE DIRECTIONS FIRST

It may sound silly, but failure to follow the directions for filling out the application is something that will eventually cause disqualification for many applicants. Before you set pen to paper read the form from beginning to end, no matter if the form has more pages than the last novel you read. Make a list of questions that may come up as you read. If you still have questions by the time you've completely read over the application you should call the personnel office and get the answers. Better to ask "How do I do this?" now than "Why was my application thrown out?" down the road.

You'd also be wise to consider asking for more than one application so that you can use a copy for practice purposes. If you can't get more than one, then copy the one you do have and use it for a practice sheet. Practice even if the application is a "simple" one-pager.

TYPEWRITER VS. HANDWRITING

Always, always, always *type* your application if this option is available. A neatly typewritten document is an eye-catcher and immediately sends the message that you care enough to go the extra mile. It also makes the reader's job easier and more pleasant and that can only be a good thing!

Sometimes typing is not an option. You may be asked to fill out a brief application on site and may not have the opportunity to take it home. If this happens then make sure you read the directions carefully, take your time writing, and print *legibly*.

Even if you are permitted to take the application home to fill it out you may be asked to complete it in your own handwriting. Some companies like to use this as an opportunity to judge your handwriting—yet another reason to read the directions! If the directions don't specify how you fill out the application then don't be shy—add this to your list of questions for that phone call you'll make to the Personnel Office.

Your application should be tidy for yet another reason—accuracy. You sure don't want the company background investigator to call up your last job and ask to speak to "Mr. Dork" instead of "Mr. York" all because she can't read your penmanship. Of course if the person investigating your background can't read what you wrote then maybe she'll take the time to call you, go over each and every item on your application that she can't read, and then rewrite it for you. And then there's the one about the Tooth Fairy . . . .

DOTTING *ALL* I'S AND T'S

Without exception, the biggest pet peeve most hiring entities express about the written applications they receive is *lack of completeness.* Amazing as it might seem, many applicants fail to simply fill in all the blanks—especially when it comes to the job history portion of the application. The job history section is not the place to forget about attention to detail. When potential employers see gaps in time on your job history they have the opportunity to use their imaginations to fill them in. Here's a few of their most likely thoughts:

- Hmmm. Wonder what this applicant did for six months after that first job. Something must've happened that she doesn't want us to know about.
- Wonder if this guy is just lazy? He can't even be bothered to follow the directions on the application that tell him to fill in *all* of the blanks. Bet he's likely to be a lazy employee.
- Wonder why he didn't mention the job we know he had one summer as a construction worker? Maybe he got fired and doesn't want us to know!

Employers have another complaint about incomplete job history sections on written applications—vague dates and times. If the application calls for the month, day, and year you started and ended a job then that is exactly what needs to appear in the appropriate blanks. That can be a daunting task if you have a lengthy employment history, but you need to come as close as possible to providing the information that is requested.

GETTING IT RIGHT

While we're on the subject of job history, there's nothing wrong with picking up the phone and calling your ex-employers to make sure that the correct information appears in this section. Nothing is more impressive than seeing a neat, complete, detailed, *accurate* listing of information. It won't take long for the person who conducts your background investigation to realize that you are serious enough about this career opportunity to take the time to verify dates and hunt up current phone numbers for old employers and co-workers. You've made their job a breeze and as a result you'll see the right ears come to a point in your hiring process.

Leaving other blanks in your application can prove equally as risky as leaving gaps in your job history. For example, most applications ask for references. Of course you'll want to list the people who know you best and who can give you glowing recommendations. No matter how much your friends may want to glow for you, however, they won't be able to help much if you don't list *daytime* phone numbers where they can be reached. Most personnel specialists work during traditional daytime office hours. Listing a home number for your personal reference who is never at home during the day is not going to win brownie points for your application.

WINDING UP

Even after these tips there's probably a few of you left who still feel the pressures of competition. This last piece of advice from a personnel specialist who helped hire the 250 workers mentioned at the beginning of this chapter is for you. "Do the best job you can on the written application. The truth is, if you turn in an application that has plenty of detail, is filled out completely, and leaves no stone unturned, then you are already ahead of half of the people who apply for this job."

The following page presents a sample Employment Application from Metro-Dade County (which covers metropolitan Miami, Florida) to give you an idea of the type of information you'll be asked to provide when you apply for a job as a bus operator.

PERSONNEL DEPARTMENT
PERSONNEL SERVICES DIVISION
140 WEST FLAGLER STREET · SUITE 105
MIAMI, FLORIDA 33130

EMPLOYMENT APPLICATION
JOB INFORMATION HOTLINE 375-1871   HEARING IMPAIRED CALL TDD-TTY 375-5645

DES EQUAL ACCESS OPPORTUNITY IN EMPLOYMENT AND SERVICES FOR MINORITIES / FEMALES / APPLICANTS WITH DISABILITIES

PLEASE PRINT · DO NOT WRITE IN SHADED AREAS

① SOCIAL SECURITY NUMBER

_ _ _ | _ _ | _ _ _ _

DATE ACCEPTED

FIRST NAME		MIDDLE INITIAL

POSITIONS APPLIED FOR

CITY	STATE	ZIP CODE

WORK PHONE #

TITLE _____ OCC CODE _____ DATE _____ (Q) (DNQ)   TITLE _____ OCC CODE _____ DATE _____ (Q) (DNQ)

concerning ethnicity, sex, age and disability
only, consistent with and pursuant to its
rs to these questions are voluntary, and will

ARE YOU CURRENTLY A COUNTY EMPLOYEE? (Yes)   (No)

TITLE _____ OCC CODE _____ DATE _____ (Q) (DNQ)   TITLE _____ OCC CODE _____ DATE _____ (Q) (DNQ)

FEMALE (F)

IN THE PAST FIVE YEARS, HAVE YOU BEEN CONVICTED OF A FELONY? (Yes)   (No)

TITLE _____ OCC CODE _____ DATE _____ (Q) (DNQ)   TITLE _____ OCC CODE _____ DATE _____ (Q) (DNQ)

ANT TO BE IDENTIFIED

ARE YOU A VETERAN OF THE UNITED STATES ARMED FORCES?
(B) BLACK / NON HISPANIC
(D) ASIAN OR PACIFIC ISLANDER
NATIVE

(Yes)   (No)   (IF YES, ATTACH DD214)

FROM _____ TO _____

TITLE _____ OCC CODE _____ DATE _____ (Q) (DNQ)   TITLE _____ OCC CODE _____ DATE _____ (Q) (DNQ)

ER LICENSE

VETERAN'S PREFERENCE   (NONE)   (5 PTS)   (10PTS)   (30%DIS)

TITLE _____ OCC CODE _____ DATE _____ (Q) (DNQ)   TITLE _____ OCC CODE _____ DATE _____ (Q) (DNQ)

UFFEUR'S
SS D   ☐ COMMERCIAL CLASS

LANGUAGES OTHER THAN ENGLISH _____

TITLE _____ OCC CODE _____ DATE _____ (Q) (DNQ)   TITLE _____ OCC CODE _____ DATE _____ (Q) (DNQ)

ED?   (Yes)   (No)

CERTIFICATIONS / LICENSES _____

TITLE _____ OCC CODE _____ DATE _____ (Q) (DNQ)   TITLE _____ OCC CODE _____ DATE _____ (Q) (DNQ)

EDUCATION

	DATES OF ATTENDANCE		SEMESTER OR CREDIT HOURS (NUMBER)	COURSE TITLES OR MAJOR FIELD	DEGREE OR CERTIFICATE RECEIVED
ELOCATED and source	FROM	TO			

EMPLOYMENT RECORD

LIST PREVIOUS EMPLOYMENT HISTORY. START WITH YOUR PRESENT EMPLOYMENT, OR IF UNEMPLOYED, YOUR MOST RECENT EMPLOYMENT, AND LIST YOUR WORK RECORD IN REVERSE ORDER. IF YOU HAVE HELD MORE THAN ONE POSITION WITH THE SAME ORGANIZATION, LIST EACH POSITION AS A SEPARATE PERIOD OF EMPLOYMENT. BE SURE TO SHOW WHERE EMPLOYMENT MAY BE VERIFIED. INCLUDE VOLUNTEER AND PAID TEMPORARY OR PART-TIME WORK AND MILITARY EXPERIENCE.

TYPE

MOST RECENT JOB _____ EMPLOYER _____ ADDRESS _____ PHONE # _____

FROM _____ TO _____ JOB TITLE _____ SUPERVISOR'S NAME _____

DESCRIBE YOUR WORK _____

2nd MOST RECENT JOB _____ EMPLOYER _____ ADDRESS _____ PHONE # _____

FROM _____ TO _____ JOB TITLE _____ SUPERVISOR'S NAME _____

DESCRIBE YOUR WORK _____

3RD MOST RECENT JOB _____ EMPLOYER _____ ADDRESS _____ PHONE # _____

FROM _____ TO _____ JOB TITLE _____ SUPERVISOR'S NAME _____

DESCRIBE YOUR WORK _____

4TH MOST RECENT JOB _____ EMPLOYER _____ ADDRESS _____ PHONE # _____

FROM _____ TO _____ JOB TITLE _____ SUPERVISOR'S NAME _____

DESCRIBE YOUR WORK _____

IT IS THE POLICY OF METROPOLITAN DADE COUNTY THAT HIRING DECISIONS WILL BE MADE CONTINGENT UPON THE RESULTS OF A PHYSICAL EXAMINATION, INCLUDING ALCOHOL AND DRUG SCREENING, PRIOR TO EMPLOYMENT. YOUR FINGERPRINTS WILL BE TAKEN FOR ROUTINE CHECK.

CERTIFICATION: I hereby certify that all statements made on this form are true to the best of my knowledge. I realize that should an investigation disclose any misrepresentation, I may be subject to dismissal. In accordance with the provisions of Ordinance No. 77-39, I hereby certify that I am presently a resident of Dade County, or if not a resident, I hereby agree to establish my residence within Dade County within (6) six months of employment by the County, I further understand that my failure to comply with the provisions of said ordinance may result in my automatic termination from County employment.

Date _____ Signature _____

METRO DADE

C·H·A·P·T·E·R

EASYSMART TEST PREPARATION SYSTEM

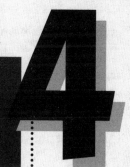

CHAPTER SUMMARY

Taking a Sanitation Worker Exam can be tough. It demands a lot of preparation if you want to achieve a top score. If your city uses your written exam score to determine your rank on the eligibility list, your chances of being hired depend on how well you do on the exam. The EasySmart Test Preparation System, developed exclusively for LearningExpress by leading test experts, gives you the discipline and attitude you need to be a winner.

First, the bad news: Taking the Sanitation Worker Exam is no picnic, and neither is getting ready for it. Your future career as a sanitation worker depends on your getting a high score, but there are all sorts of pitfalls that can keep you from doing your best on this all-important exam. Here are some of the obstacles that can stand in the way of your success:

- Being unfamiliar with the format of the exam
- Being paralyzed by test anxiety
- Leaving your preparation to the last minute
- Not preparing at all!
- Not knowing vital test-taking skills: how to pace yourself through the exam, how to use the process of elimination, and when to guess

- Not being in tip-top mental and physical shape
- Messing up on test day by arriving late at the test site, having to work on an empty stomach, or shivering through the exam because the room is cold

What's the common denominator in all these test-taking pitfalls? One word: *control*. Who's in control, you or the exam?

Now the good news: The EasySmart Test Preparation System puts *you* in control. In just nine easy-to-follow steps, you will learn everything you need to know to make sure that *you* are in charge of your preparation and your performance on the exam. *Other* test-takers may let the test get the better of them; *other* test-takers may be unprepared or out of shape, but not *you*. *You* will have taken all the steps you need to take to get a high score on the Sanitation Worker Exam.

Here's how the EasySmart Test Preparation System works: Nine easy steps lead you through everything you need to know and do to get ready to master your exam. Each of the steps listed below includes both reading about the step and one or more activities. It's important that you do the activities along with the reading, or you won't be getting the full benefit of the system. Each step tells you approximately how much time that step will take you to complete.

Step 1. Get Information	60 minutes
Step 2. Conquer Test Anxiety	20 minutes
Step 3. Make a Plan	25 minutes
Step 4. Learn to Manage Your Time	10 minutes
Step 5. Learn to Use the Process of Elimination	20 minutes
Step 6. Know When to Guess	20 minutes
Step 7. Reach Your Peak Performance Zone	10 minutes
Step 8. Get Your Act Together	10 minutes
Step 9. Do It!	5 minutes
Total	**3 hours**

We estimate that working through the entire system will take you approximately three hours, though it's perfectly OK if you work faster or slower than the time estimates assume. If you can take a whole afternoon or evening, you can work through the whole EasySmart Test Preparation System in one sitting. Otherwise, you can break it up, and do just one or two steps a day for the next several days. It's up to you—remember, *you're* in control.

STEP 1: GET INFORMATION

Time to complete: 60 minutes
Activities: Use the suggestions listed here to find out about the content of your exam.

Knowledge is power. The first step in the EasySmart Test Preparation System is finding out everything you can about the Sanitation Worker Exam. Once you have your information, the next steps in the EasySmart Test Preparation System will show you what to do about it.

Part A: Straight Talk About Civil Service Exams

Why do you have to take this exam, anyway? The fact is that way too many people want a secure job with the city, far more than can ever be hired—far more, in fact, than the city can even afford to process in a conventional application-resume-interview process. The city needs a way to dramatically cut the number of applicants they have to consider. That's where the exam comes in.

Like any civil service test, the Sanitation Worker Exam is a screening device. It enables the city to rank candidates according to their exam score and then to pull only from the top of that list to get applicants to go through the rest of the selection process. Since the exam assesses job-related skills—abilities you actually have to have to be a good sanitation worker—there's a rough correlation between how well a person does on the test and how good an employee that person will make. But it's only a rough correlation. There are all sorts of things a written exam like this can't test: whether you can get along with the public, fellow employees, and supervisors; whether you're likely to show up on time or call in sick a lot; and so on. But those kinds of things are hard to evaluate, while whether or not you fill in the right circle on a bubble answer sheet is easy to evaluate. So most cities use an exam simply to cut the number of applicants they have to deal with.

This information should help you keep some perspective on the exam and what it means. Don't make the mistake of thinking that your score determines who you are or how smart you are or whether you'll make a good employee, with the city or elsewhere. All it shows is whether you can fill in the little circles correctly. Of course, whether you can fill in the little circles correctly is still vitally important to you! After all, your chances of being hired depend on your getting a top score. And that's why you're here—using the EasySmart Test Preparation System to achieve control over your exam.

Part B: What's on the Test

If you haven't already done so, stop here and read the first three chapters of this book, which give you vital information on becoming a sanitation worker, hiring procedures for major U.S. cities, and filling out a civil service application.

Sanitation worker exams vary from city to city. Most test the skills in the practice exams in this book—reading, verbal expression (writing), judgment and common sense, spatial relations and map reading, and sometimes math. Some exams, however, are given in a different format—and you need to know what *your* exam will be like.

How best to get that information also varies from city to city. Here are some avenues to try:

- **Go to the public library,** which may have information on jobs available in your city. Ask the librarian at the reference desk for help.
- **Call the Sanitaion Department,** Department of Public Works, or whatever it's called in your city. You can find the number in the blue (government) pages of your phone book.
- **Call the city's Department of Personnel.** This department may be called "Civil Service" or "Human Resources." This number is also in the blue pages of the phone book, or you may be referred to this department by the Sanitation Department.
- **Ask around.** Friends or relatives who already work for the city—better yet, for the Bus Department—may have inside information that hasn't yet been released to the public.

If an exam has been scheduled in your city, or if your city conducts ongoing exams, one of these steps should give you an exam announcement or similar document that outlines the content of your test. If no exam is scheduled, you may simply have to wait—and put your name on a notification list, if the department keeps one. In the meantime, however, you can still go through the rest of the steps in the EasySmart Test Preparation System and work through the rest of this book, to make sure you're prepared when the exam is announced.

STEP 2: CONQUER TEST ANXIETY

Time to complete: 20 minutes
Activity: Take the Test Stress Test
Having complete information about the exam is the first step in getting control of the exam. Next, you have to overcome one of the biggest obstacles to test success: test anxiety. Test anxiety can not only impair your performance on the exam itself; it can even keep you from preparing! In Step 2, you'll learn stress management techniques that will help you succeed on your exam. Learn these strategies now, and practice them as you work through the exams in this book, so they'll be second nature to you by exam day.

COMBATING TEST ANXIETY
The first thing you need to know is that a little test anxiety is a good thing. Everyone gets nervous before a big exam—and if that nervousness motivates you to prepare thoroughly, so much the better. It's said that Sir Laurence Olivier, one of the foremost British actors of this century, threw up before every performance. His stage fright didn't impair his performance; in fact, it probably gave him a little extra edge—just the kind of edge you need to do well, whether on a stage or in an examination room.

On the next page is the Test Stress Test. Stop here and answer the questions on that page, to find out whether your level of test anxiety is something you should worry about.

Test Stress Test

You only need to worry about test anxiety if it is extreme enough to impair your performance. The following questionnaire will provide a diagnosis of your level of test anxiety. In the blank before each statement, write the number that most accurately describes your experience.

0 = Never   1 = Once or twice   2 = Sometimes   3 = Often

_____ I have gotten so nervous before an exam that I simply put down the books and didn't study for it.

_____ I have experienced disabling physical symptoms such as vomiting and severe headaches because I was nervous about an exam.

_____ I have simply not showed up for an exam because I was scared to take it.

_____ I have experienced dizziness and disorientation while taking an exam.

_____ I have had trouble filling in the little circles because my hands were shaking too hard.

_____ I have failed an exam because I was too nervous to complete it.

_____ **Total: Add up the numbers in the blanks above.**

Your Test Stress Score

Here are the steps you should take, depending on your score. If you scored:

- **Below 3,** your level of test anxiety is nothing to worry about; it's probably just enough to give you that little extra edge.
- **Between 3 and 6,** your test anxiety may be enough to impair your performance, and you should practice the stress management techniques listed in this section to try to bring your test anxiety down to manageable levels.
- **Above 6,** your level of test anxiety is a serious concern. In addition to practicing the stress management techniques listed in this section, you may want to seek additional, personal help. Call your local high school or community college and ask for the academic counselor. Tell the counselor that you have a level of test anxiety that sometimes keeps you from being able to take the exam. The counselor may be willing to help you or may suggest someone else you should talk to.

Stress Management Before the Test

If you feel your level of anxiety getting the best of you in the weeks before the test, here is what you need to do to bring the level down again:

- **Get prepared.** There's nothing like knowing what to expect and being prepared for it to put you in control of test anxiety. That's why you're reading this book. Use it faithfully, and remind yourself that you're better prepared than most of the people taking the test.

- **Practice self-confidence.** A positive attitude is a great way to combat test anxiety. This is no time to be humble or shy. Stand in front of the mirror and say to your reflection, "I'm prepared. I'm full of self-confidence. I'm going to ace this test. I know I can do it." Say it into a tape recorder and play it back once a day. If you hear it often enough, you'll believe it.

- **Fight negative messages.** Every time someone starts telling you how hard the exam is or how it's almost impossible to get a high score, start telling them your self-confidence messages above. If the someone with the negative messages is *you*, telling yourself *you don't do well on exams, you just can't do this,* don't listen. Turn on your tape recorder and listen to your self-confidence messages.

- **Visualize.** Imagine yourself driving your collection route as a city sanitation worker. Think of yourself coming home with your first paycheck as a city employee and taking your family or friends out to celebrate. Visualizing success can help make it happen—and it reminds you of why you're going to all this work in preparing for the exam.

- **Exercise.** Physical activity helps calm your body down and focus your mind. Besides, being in good physical shape can actually help you do well on the exam. Go for a run, lift weights, go swimming—and do it regularly.

Stress Management on Test Day

There are several ways you can bring down your level of test anxiety on test day. They'll work best if you practice them in the weeks before the test, so you know which ones work best for you.

- **Deep breathing.** Take a deep breath while you count to five. Hold it for a count of one, then let it out on a count of five. Repeat several times.

- **Move your body.** Try rolling your head in a circle. Rotate your shoulders. Shake your hands from the wrist. Many people find these movements very relaxing.

- **Visualize again.** Think of the place where you are most relaxed: lying on the beach in the sun, walking through the park, or whatever. Now close your eyes and imagine you're actually there. If you practice in advance, you'll find that you only need a few seconds of this exercise to experience a significant increase in your sense of well-being.

When anxiety threatens to overwhelm you right there during the exam, there are still things you can do to manage the stress level:

- **Repeat your self-confidence messages.** You should have them memorized by now. Say them quietly to yourself, and believe them!
- **Visualize one more time.** This time, visualize yourself moving smoothly and quickly through the test answering every question right and finishing just before time is up. Like most visualization techniques, this one works best if you've practiced it ahead of time.
- **Find an easy question.** Skim over the test until you find an easy question, and answer it. Getting even one circle filled in gets you into the test-taking groove.
- **Take a mental break.** Everyone loses concentration once in a while during a long test. It's normal, so you shouldn't worry about it. Instead, accept what has happened. Say to yourself, "Hey, I lost it there for a minute. My brain is taking a break." Put down your pencil, close your eyes, and do some deep breathing for a few seconds. Then you're ready to go back to work.

Try these techniques ahead of time, and see if they don't work for you!

STEP 3: MAKE A PLAN

Time to complete: 25 minutes
Activity: Construct a study plan
Maybe the most important thing you can do to get control of yourself and your exam is to make a study plan. Too many people fail to prepare simply because they fail to plan. Spending hours on the day before the exam poring over sample test questions not only raises your level of test anxiety, it also is simply no substitute for careful preparation and practice over time.

Don't fall into the cram trap. Take control of your preparation time by mapping out a study schedule. On the following pages are four sample schedules, based on the amount of time you have before the Sanitation Worker Exam. If you're the kind of person who needs deadlines and assignments to motivate you for a project, here they are. If you're the kind of person who doesn't like to follow other people's plans, you can use the suggested schedules here to construct your own.

Even more important than making a plan is making a commitment. You can't improve your reading and judgment skills overnight. You have to set aside some time every day for study and practice. Try for at least 20 minutes a day. Twenty minutes daily will do you much more good than two hours on Saturday.

If you have months before the exam, you're lucky. Don't put off your study until the week before the exam. Start now. A few minutes a day, with half an hour or more on weekends, can make a big difference in your score—and in your chances of getting the job!

SCHEDULE A: THE LEISURE PLAN

If you have six months or more in which to prepare, you're lucky! Make the most of your time.

Time	Preparation
Exam minus 6 months	Take the first practice exam in Chapter 5. Use your score to help you decide on <u>one</u> area to concentrate on this month, and read the corresponding chapter. When you get to that chapter in this plan, review it.
Exam minus 5 months	Read Chapter 6 and work through the exercises. Set aside some time every day for some serious reading—books and magazines, not comic books. Find other people who are preparing for the test and form a study group.
Exam minus 4 months	Read Chapters 7 and 8 and work through the exercises. You're still doing your reading aren't you?
Exam minus 3 months	Read Chapter 9 and work through the exercises. Watch real sanitation workers in action to see how they handle difficult situations.
Exam minus 2 months	Read Chapter 10 and work through the exercises. Practice your math skills in everyday situations.
Exam minus 1 month	Take the second practice test in Chapter 11. Use your score to help you decide where to concentrate your efforts. Review the relevant chapters, and get the help of a friend or teacher.
Exam minus 1 week	Take the third practice test, and again review the areas that give you the most trouble.
Exam minus 1 day	Relax. Do something unrelated to the exam. Eat a good meal and go to bed at your usual time.

SCHEDULE B: THE JUST-ENOUGH-TIME PLAN

If you have three to five months before the exam, that should be enough time to prepare for the written test. This schedule assumes four months; stretch it out or compress it if you have more or less time.

Time	Preparation
Exam minus 4 months	Take the first practice test in Chapter 5. Then read Chapter 6 and work through the exercises. Start a program of serious reading to improve your reading comprehension.
Exam minus 3 months	Read Chapters 7 and 8 and work through the exercises. Form a study group with other people who are preparing for the exam.
Exam minus 2 months	Read Chapters 9 and 10 and work through the exercises. Watch real sanitation workers to see how they handle difficult situations, and work on your math skills in everyday situations.
Exam minus 1 month	Take the second practice test in Chapter 11. Use your score to help you decide where to concentrate your efforts this month. Review the relevant chapters, and get the help of a friend or teacher.
Exam minus 1 week	Take the third practice test. See how much you've learned in the past months? Review the chapter on the <u>one</u> area that gives you the most trouble.
Exam minus 1 day	Relax. Do something unrelated to the exam. Eat a good meal and go to bed at your usual time.

SCHEDULE C: MORE STUDY IN LESS TIME

If you have one to three months before the exam, you still have enough time for some concentrated study that will help you improve your score. This schedule is built around a two-month timeframe. If you have only one month, spend an extra couple of hours a week to get all these steps in. If you have three months, take some of the steps from Schedule B and fit them in.

Time	Preparation
Exam minus 8 weeks	Take the first practice test in Chapter 5. Evaluate your performance to find one or two areas you're weakest in. Choose one or two chapter(s) from among Chapters 6–10 to read in these two weeks. When you get to those chapters in this plan, review them.
Exam minus 6 weeks	Read Chapters 6 and 7 and work through the exercises.
Exam minus 4 weeks	Read Chapters 8, 9, and 10 and work through the exercises.
Exam minus 2 weeks	Take the second practice test in Chapter 11. Then score it and read the answer explanations until you're sure you understand them. Review the areas where your score is lowest.
Exam minus 1 week	Take the third practice test in Chapter 12. Review Chapters 6–10, concentrating on the areas where a little work can help the most.
Exam minus 1 day	Relax. Do something unrelated to the exam. Eat a good meal and go to bed at your usual time.

SCHEDULE D: THE CRAM PLAN

If you have three weeks or less before the exam, you really have your work cut out for you. Carve half an hour out of your day, *every day,* for study. This schedule assumes you have the whole three weeks to prepare in; if you have less time, you'll have to compress the schedule accordingly.

Time	Preparation
Exam minus 3 weeks	Take the first practice test in Chapter 5. Read Chapters 6 and 7 and work through the exercises.
Exam minus 2 weeks	Read Chapters 8, 9, and 10 and work through the exercises. Take the second practice test in Chapter 11.
Exam minus 1 week	Take the third practice test in Chapter 12. Evaluate your performance on the second and third practice tests. Review the parts of Chapters 6–10 that you had the most trouble with. Get a friend or teacher to help you with the section you had the most difficulty with.
Exam minus 2 days	Review all three tests. Make sure you understand the answer explanations.
Exam minus 1 day	Relax. Do something unrelated to the exam. Eat a good meal and go to bed at your usual time.

STEP 4: LEARN TO MANAGE YOUR TIME

Time to complete: 10 minutes to read, many hours of practice!

Activities: Practice these strategies as you take the sample tests in this book

Steps 4, 5, and 6 of the EasySmart Test Preparation System put you in charge of your exam by showing you test-taking strategies that work. Practice these strategies as you take the sample tests in this book, and then you'll be ready to use them on test day.

First, you'll take control of your time on the exam. Most civil service exams have a time limit, which may give you more than enough time to complete all the questions—or may not. It's a terrible feeling to hear the examiner say, "Five minutes left," when you're only three-quarters of the way through the test. Here are some tips to keep that from happening to *you*.

- **Follow directions.** If the directions are given orally, listen to them. If they're written on the exam booklet, read them carefully. Ask questions *before* the exam begins if there's anything you don't understand. If you're allowed to write in your exam booklet, write down the beginning time and the ending time of the exam.
- **Pace yourself.** Glance at your watch every ten or fifteen minutes, and compare the time to how far you've gotten in the exam. When one-quarter of the time has elapsed, you should be a quarter of the way through the exam, and so on. If you're falling behind, pick up the pace a bit.
- **Keep moving.** Don't dither around on one question. If you don't know the answer, skip the question and move on. Circle the number of the question in your test booklet in case you have time to come back to it later.
- **Keep track of your place on the answer sheet.** If you skip a question, make sure you skip on the answer sheet too. Check yourself every 5–10 questions to make sure the question number and the answer sheet number are still the same.
- **Don't rush.** Though you should keep moving, rushing won't help. Try to keep calm and work methodically and quickly.

STEP 5: LEARN TO USE THE PROCESS OF ELIMINATION

Time to complete: 20 minutes

Activity: Complete worksheet on Using the Process of Elimination

After time management, your next most important tool for taking control of your exam is using the process of elimination wisely. It's standard test-taking wisdom that you should always read all the answer choices before choosing your answer. This helps you find the right answer by eliminating wrong answer choices. And, sure enough, that standard wisdom applies to your exam, too.

Let's say you're facing a vocabulary question that goes like this:

13. "Biology uses a <u>binomial</u> system of classification." In this sentence, the word <u>binomial</u> most nearly means
   a. understanding the law
   b. having two names
   c. scientifically sound
   d. having a double meaning

If you happen to know what *binomial* means, of course, you don't need to use the process of elimination, but let's assume that, like most people, you don't. So you look at the answer choices. "Understanding the law" sure doesn't sound very likely for something having to do with biology. So you eliminate choice **a**—and now you only have three answer choices to deal with. Mark an X next to choice **a** so you never have to read it again.

On to the other answer choices. If you know that the prefix *bi-* means *two*, as in *bicycle*, you'll flag answer **b** as a possible answer. Mark a check mark beside it, meaning "good answer, I might use this one."

Choice **c,** "scientifically sound," is a possibility. At least it's about science, not law. It could work here, though, when you think about it, having a "scientifically sound" classification system in a scientific field is kind of redundant. You remember the *bi* thing in *binomial,* and probably continue to like answer **b** better. But you're not sure, so you put a question mark next to **c,** meaning "well, maybe."

Now, choice **d,** "having a double meaning." You're still keeping in mind that *bi-* means *two,* so this one looks possible at first. But then you look again at the sentence the word belongs in, and you think, "Why would biology want a system of classification that has two meanings? That wouldn't work very well!" If you're really taken with the idea that *bi* means *two,* you might put a question mark here. But if you're feeling a little more confident, you'll put an X. You've already got a better answer picked out.

Now your question looks like this:

13. "Biology uses a <u>binomial</u> system of classification." In this sentence, the word <u>binomial</u> most nearly means
   × **a.** understanding the law
   ✔ **b.** having two names
   ? **c.** scientifically sound
   ? **d.** having a double meaning

You've got just one check mark, for a good answer. If you're pressed for time, you should simply mark answer **b** on your answer sheet. If you've got the time to be extra careful, you could compare your check-mark answer to your question-mark answers to make sure that it's better. (It is: the *binomial* system in biology is the one that gives a two-part genus and species name like *homo sapiens.*)

It's good to have a system for marking good, bad, and maybe answers. We're recommending this one:

   × = bad
   ✔ = good
   ? = maybe

If you don't like these marks, devise your own system. Just make sure you do it long before test day—while you're working through the practice exams in this book—so you won't have to worry about it during the test.

Even when you think you're absolutely clueless about a question, you can often use process of elimination to get rid of one answer choice. If so, you're better prepared to make an educated guess, as you'll see in Step 6. More often, the process of elimination allows you to get down to only *two* possibly right answers. Then you're in a strong position to guess. And sometimes, even though you don't know the right answer, you find it simply by getting rid of the wrong ones, as you did in the example above.

Try using your powers of elimination on the questions in the worksheet Using the Process of Elimination beginning on this page. The answer explanations there show one possible way you might use the process to arrive at the right answer.

The process of elimination is your tool for the next step, which is knowing when to guess.

Using the Process of Elimination

Use the process of elimination to answer the following questions. (These questions are extra difficult to force you to use elimination. Don't worry; the questions on your exam won't be this hard!)

1. Ilsa is as old as Meghan will be in five years. The difference between Ed's age and Meghan's age is twice the difference between Ilsa's age and Meghan's age. Ed is 29. How old is Ilsa?
   a. 4
   b. 10
   c. 19
   d. 24

2. "All drivers of commercial vehicles must carry a valid commercial driver's license whenever operating a commercial vehicle." According to this sentence, which of the following people need NOT carry a commercial driver's license?
   a. a truck driver idling his engine while waiting to be directed to a loading dock
   b. a sanitation worker backing her bus out of the way of another bus in the bus lot
   c. a taxi driver driving his personal car to the grocery store
   d. a limousine driver taking the limousine to her home after dropping off her last passenger of the evening

3. Smoking tobacco has been linked to
   a. increased risk of stroke and heart attack
   b. all forms of respiratory disease
   c. increasing mortality rates over the past ten years
   d. juvenile delinquency

---

4. Which of the following words is spelled correctly?
   a. incorrigible
   b. outragous
   c. domestickated
   d. understandible

Answers

Here are the answers, as well as some suggestions as to how you might have used the process of elimination to find them.

1. **d.** You should have eliminated answer **a** off the bat. Ilsa can't be four years old if Meghan is going to be Ilsa's age in five years. The best way to eliminate other answer choices is to try plugging them in to the information given in the problem. For instance, for answer **b,** if Ilsa is 10, then Meghan must be 5. The difference in their ages is 5. The difference between Ed's age, 29, and Meghan's age, 5, is 24. Is 24 two times 5? No. Then answer **b** is wrong. You could eliminate answer **c** in the same way and be left with answer **d.**

2. **c.** Note the word *not* in the question, and go through the answers one by one. Is the truck driver in choice **a** "operating a commericial vehicle"? Yes, idling counts as "operating," so he needs to have a commercial driver's license. Likewise, the sanitation worker in answer **b** is operating a commercial vehicle; the question doesn't say the operator has to be on the street. The limo driver in **d** is operating a commercial vehicle, even if it doesn't have passenger in it. However, the cabbie in answer **c** is *not* operating a commercial vehicle, but his own private car.

3. **a.** You could eliminate answer **b** simply because of the presence of the word *all*. Such absolutes hardly ever appear in correct answer choices. Choice **c** looks attractive until you think a little about what you know—aren't *fewer* people smoking these days, rather than more? So how could smoking be responsible for a higher mortality rate? (If you didn't know that *mortality rate* means the rate at which people die, you might keep this choice as a possibility, but you'd still be able to eliminate two answers and have only two to choose from.) And choice **d** is plain silly, so you could eliminate that one, too. And you're left with the correct choice, **a.**

4. **a.** How you used the process of elimination here depends on which words you recognized as being spelled incorrectly. If you knew that the correct spellings were *outrageous, domesticated,* and *understandable,* then you were home free. Surely you knew that at least one of those words was wrong!

STEP 6: KNOW WHEN TO GUESS

Time to complete: 20 minutes

Activity: Complete worksheet on Your Guessing Ability

Armed with the process of elimination, you're ready to take control of one of the big questions in test-taking: Should I guess? The first and main answer is Yes. Unless the exam has a so-called "guessing penalty," you have nothing to lose and everything to gain from guessing. The more complicated answer depends both on the exam and on you—your personality and your "guessing intuition."

Most civil service exams don't use a guessing penalty. The number of questions you answer correctly yields your score, and there's no penalty for wrong answers. So most of the time, you don't have to worry—simply go ahead and guess. But if you find that your exam does have a "guessing penalty," you should read the section below to find out what that means to you.

How the "Guessing Penalty" Works

A "guessing penalty" really only works against *random* guessing—filling in the little circles to make a nice pattern on your answer sheet. If you can eliminate one or more answer choices, as outlined above, you're better off taking a guess than leaving the answer blank, even on the sections that have a penalty.

Here's how a "guessing penalty" works: Depending on the number of answer choices in a given exam, some proportion of the number of questions you get wrong is subtracted from the total number of questions you got right. For instance, if there are four answer choices, typically the "guessing penalty" is one-third of your wrong answers. Suppose you took a test of 100 questions. You answered 88 of them right and 12 wrong.

If there's no guessing penalty, your score is simply 88. But if there's a one-third point guessing penalty, the scorers take your 12 wrong answers and divide by 3 to come up with 4. Then they *subtract* that 4 from your correct-answer score of 88 to leave you with a score of 84. Thus, you would have been better off if you had simply not answered those 12 questions that you weren't sure of. Then your total score would still be 88, because there wouldn't be anything to subtract.

What You Should Do About the Guessing Penalty

That's how a guessing penalty works. The first thing this means for you is that marking your answer sheet at random doesn't pay. If you're running out of time on an exam that has a guessing penalty, you should not use your remaining seconds to mark a pretty pattern on your answer sheet. Take those few seconds to try to answer one more question right.

But as soon as you get out of the realm of random guessing, the "guessing penalty" no longer works against you. If you can use the process of elimination to get rid of even one wrong answer choice, the odds stop being against you and start working in your favor.

Sticking with our example of an exam that has four answer choices, eliminating just one wrong answer makes your odds of choosing the correct answer one in three. That's the same as the one-out-of-three guessing

(continued on page 20)

Your Guessing Ability

The following are ten really hard questions. You're not supposed to know the answers. Rather, this is an assessment of your ability to guess when you don't have a clue. Read each question carefully, just as if you did expect to answer it. If you have any knowledge at all of the subject of the question, use that knowledge to help you eliminate wrong answer choices. Use this answer grid to fill in your answers to the questions.

ANSWER GRID

```
1.  Ⓐ Ⓑ Ⓒ Ⓓ        5.  Ⓐ Ⓑ Ⓒ Ⓓ        9.  Ⓐ Ⓑ Ⓒ Ⓓ
2.  Ⓐ Ⓑ Ⓒ Ⓓ        6.  Ⓐ Ⓑ Ⓒ Ⓓ       10.  Ⓐ Ⓑ Ⓒ Ⓓ
3.  Ⓐ Ⓑ Ⓒ Ⓓ        7.  Ⓐ Ⓑ Ⓒ Ⓓ
4.  Ⓐ Ⓑ Ⓒ Ⓓ        8.  Ⓐ Ⓑ Ⓒ Ⓓ
```

1. September 7 is Independence Day in
   A. India
   B. Costa Rica
   C. Brazil
   D. Australia

2. Which of the following is the formula for determining the momentum of an object?
   A. $p = mv$
   B. $F = ma$
   C. $P = IV$
   D. $E = mc^2$

3. Because of the expansion of the universe, the stars and other celestial bodies are all moving away from each other. This phenomenon is known as
   A. Newton's first law
   B. the big bang
   C. gravitational collapse
   D. Hubble flow

4. American author Gertrude Stein was born in
   A. 1713
   B. 1830
   C. 1874
   D. 1901

5. Which of the following is NOT one of the Five Classics attributed to Confucius?
   A. the I Ching
   B. the Book of Holiness
   C. the Spring and Autumn Annals
   D. the Book of History

6. The religious and philosophical doctrine that holds that the universe is constantly in a struggle between good and evil is known as
   A. Pelagianism
   B. Manichaeanism
   C. neo-Hegelianism
   D. Epicureanism

7. The third Chief Justice of the U.S. Supreme Court was
   A. John Blair
   B. William Cushing
   C. James Wilson
   D. John Jay

8. Which of the following is the poisonous portion of a daffodil?
   A. the bulb
   B. the leaves
   C. the stem
   D. the flowers

9. The winner of the Masters golf tournament in 1953 was
   A. Sam Snead
   B. Cary Middlecoff
   C. Arnold Palmer
   D. Ben Hogan

10. The state with the highest per capita personal income in 1980 was
    A. Alaska
    B. Connecticut
    C. New York
    D. Texas

Answers

Check your answers against the correct answers below.

1. C.	**5.** B.	**9.** D.
2. A.	**6.** B.	**10.** A.
3. D.	**7.** B.	
4. C.	**8.** A.	

How Did You Do?

You may have simply gotten lucky and actually known the answer to one or two questions. In addition, your guessing was more successful if you were able to use the process of elimination on any of the questions. Maybe you didn't know who the third Chief Justice was (question 7), but you knew that John Jay was the first. In that case, you would have eliminated answer **D** and therefore improved your odds of guessing right from one in four to one in three.

According to probability, you should get 2 1/2 answers correct, so getting either two or three right would be average. If you got four or more right, you may be a really terrific guesser. If you got one or none right, you may be a really bad guesser.

Keep in mind, though, that this is only a small sample. You should continue to keep track of your guessing ability as you work through the sample questions in this book. Circle the numbers of questions you guess on as you make your guess; or, if you don't have time while you take the practice tests, go back afterward and try to remember which questions you guessed at. Remember, on a test with four answer choices, your chances of getting a right answer is one in four. So keep a separate "guessing" score for each exam. How many questions did you guess on? How many did you get right? If the number you got right is at least one-fourth of the number of questions you guessed on, you are at least an average guesser, maybe better—and you should always go ahead and guess on the real exam. If the number you got right is significantly lower than one-fourth of the number you guessed on, you should not guess on exams where there is a guessing penalty unless you can eliminate a wrong answer. If there's no guessing penalty you would, frankly, be safe in guessing anyway, but maybe you'd feel more comfortable if you guessed only selectively, when you can eliminate a wrong answer or at least have a good feeling about one of the answer choices.

penalty—even odds. If you eliminate two answer choices, your odds are one in two—better than the guessing penalty. In either case, you should go ahead and choose one of the remaining answer choices.

WHEN THERE IS NO GUESSING PENALTY

As noted above, most civil service exams don't have a guessing penalty. That means that, all other things being equal, you should always go ahead and guess, even if you have no idea what the question means. Nothing can happen to you if you're wrong. But all other things aren't necessarily equal. The other factor in deciding whether or not to guess, besides the exam and whether or not it has a guessing penalty, is you. There are two things you need to know about yourself before you go into the exam:

- Are you a risk-taker?
- Are you a good guesser?

Your risk-taking temperament matters most on exams with a guessing penalty. Without a guessing penalty, even if you're a play-it-safe person, guessing is perfectly safe. Overcome your anxieties, and go ahead and mark an answer.

But what if you're not much of a risk-taker, *and* you think of yourself as the world's worst guesser? Complete the worksheet Your Guessing Ability to get an idea of how good your intuition is.

STEP 7: REACH YOUR PEAK PERFORMANCE ZONE

Time to complete: 10 minutes to read; weeks to complete!
Activity: Complete the Physical Preparation Checklist
To get ready for a challenge like a big exam, you have to take control of your physical, as well as your mental, state. Exercise, proper diet, and rest will ensure that your body works with, rather than against, your mind on test day, as well as during your preparation.

EXERCISE

If you don't already have a regular exercise program going, the time during which you're preparing for an exam is actually an excellent time to start one. And if you're already keeping fit—or trying to get that way—don't let the pressure of preparing for an exam fool you into quitting now. Exercise helps reduce stress by pumping wonderful good-feeling hormones called endorphins into your system. It also increases the oxygen supply throughout your body, including your brain, so you'll be at peak performance on test day.

A half hour of vigorous activity—enough to raise a sweat—every day should be your aim. If you're really pressed for time, every other day is OK. Choose an activity you like and get out there and do it. Jogging with a friend always makes the time go faster, or take a radio.

But don't overdo. You don't want to exhaust yourself. Moderation is the key.

Physical Preparation Checklist

For the week before the test, write down 1) what physical exercise you engaged in and for how long and 2) what you ate for each meal. Remember, you're trying for at least half an hour of exercise every other day (preferably every day) and a balanced diet that's light on junk food.

Exam minus 7 days
Exercise: _____ for _____ minutes
Breakfast: _____
Lunch: _____
Dinner: _____
Snacks: _____

Exam minus 6 days
Exercise: _____ for _____ minutes
Breakfast: _____
Lunch: _____
Dinner: _____
Snacks: _____

Exam minus 5 days
Exercise: _____ for _____ minutes
Breakfast: _____
Lunch: _____
Dinner: _____
Snacks: _____

Exam minus 4 days
Exercise: _____ for _____ minutes
Breakfast: _____
Lunch: _____
Dinner: _____
Snacks: _____

Exam minus 3 days
Exercise: _____ for _____ minutes
Breakfast: _____
Lunch: _____
Dinner: _____
Snacks: _____

Exam minus 2 days

Exercise: _____ for _____ minutes

Breakfast: _____

Lunch: _____

Dinner: _____

Snacks: _____

Exam minus 1 day

Exercise: _____ for _____ minutes

Breakfast: _____

Lunch: _____

Dinner: _____

Snacks: _____

DIET

First of all, cut out the junk. Go easy on caffeine and nicotine, and eliminate alcohol and any other drugs from your system at least two weeks before the exam. Promise yourself a binge the night after the exam, if need be.

What your body needs for peak performance is simply a balanced diet. Eat plenty of fruits and vegetables, along with protein and carbohydrates. Foods that are high in lecithin (an amino acid), such as fish and beans, are especially good "brain foods."

The night before the exam, you might "carbo-load" the way athletes do before a contest. Eat a big plate of spaghetti, rice and beans, or whatever your favorite carbohydrate is.

REST

You probably know how much sleep you need every night to be at your best, even if you don't always get it. Make sure you do get that much sleep, though, for at least a week before the exam. Moderation is important here, too. Extra sleep will just make you groggy.

If you're not a morning person and your exam will be given in the morning, you should reset your internal clock so that your body doesn't think you're taking an exam at 3 a.m. You have to start this process well before the exam. The way it works is to get up half an hour earlier each morning, and then go to bed half an hour earlier that night. Don't try it the other way around; you'll just toss and turn if you go to bed early without having gotten up early. The next morning, get up another half an hour earlier, and so on. How long you will have to do this depends on how late you're used to getting up.

STEP 8: GET YOUR ACT TOGETHER

Time to complete: 10 minutes to read; time to complete will vary
Activity: Complete Final Preparations worksheet
You're in control of your mind and body; you're in charge of test anxiety, your preparation, and your test-taking strategies. Now it's time to take charge of external factors, like the testing site and the materials you need to take the exam.

FIND OUT WHERE THE TEST IS AND MAKE A TRIAL RUN

The city will notify you when and where your exam is being held. Do you know how to get to the testing site? Do you know how long it will take to get there? If not, make a trial run, preferably on the same day of the week at the same time of day. Make note, on the worksheet Final Preparations, of the amount of time it will take you to get to the exam site. Plan on arriving 10–15 minutes early so you can get the lay of the land, use the bathroom, and calm down. Then figure out how early you will have to get up that morning, and make sure you get up that early every day for a week before the exam.

GATHER YOUR MATERIALS

The night before the exam, lay out the clothes you will wear and the materials you have to bring with you to the exam. Plan on dressing in layers; you won't have any control over the temperature of the examination room. Have a sweater or jacket you can take off if it's warm. Use the checklist on the worksheet Final Preparations to help you pull together what you'll need.

Don't Skip Breakfast

Even if you don't usually eat breakfast, do so on exam morning. A cup of coffee doesn't count. Don't do doughnuts or other sweet foods, either. A sugar high will leave you with a sugar low in the middle of the exam. A mix of protein and carbohydrates is best: cereal with milk and just a little sugar, or eggs with toast, will do your body a world of good.

STEP 9: DO IT!

Time to complete: 5 minutes, plus test-taking time
Activity: Ace the Sanitation Worker Exam!
Fast forward to exam day. You're ready. You made a study plan and followed through. You practiced your test-taking strategies while working through this book. You're in control of your physical, mental, and emotional state. You know when and where to show up and what to bring with you. In other words, you're better prepared than most of the other people taking the Sanitation Worker Exam with you. You're psyched.

Just one more thing. When you're done with the Sanitation Worker exam, you will have earned a reward. Plan a celebration for exam night. Call up your friends and plan a party, or have a nice dinner for two—whatever your heart desires. Give yourself something to look forward to.

And then do it. Go into the Sanitation Worker Exam, full of confidence, armed with test-taking strategies you've practiced till they're second nature. You're in control of yourself, your environment, and your performance on the exam. You're ready to succeed. So do it. Go in there and ace the exam. And look forward to your future career as a sanitation worker!

Final Preparations

Getting to the Exam Site

Location of exam: _____

Date of exam: _____

Time of exam: _____

Do I know how to get to the exam site? Yes _____ No _____
If no, make a trial run.

Time it will take to get to exam site: _____

Things to lay out the night before the exam

Clothes I will wear   _____

Sweater/jacket   _____

Watch   _____

Admission card   _____

Photo ID   _____

4 No. 2. pencils   _____

_____   _____

_____   _____

C·H·A·P·T·E·R

SANITATION WORKER PRACTICE EXAM 1

5

CHAPTER SUMMARY

This is the first of three practice exams in this book based on the most commonly tested areas on sanitation worker written exams nationwide. Use this test to see how you would do if you had to take the exam today.

The exam that follows covers the skills most often included on written sanitation worker exams across the country. Since exams do vary from city to city, you may find some differences between this practice exam and the real thing. However, the skills tested here have been tested in the past and are very important for the actual work of a sanitation worker, so this exam will provide vital practice.

The practice exam consists of 70 multiple-choice questions in the following areas: understanding written language; communicating information; using judgment to recognize a problem; following rules; using spatial reasoning; and adding, subtracting, multiplying, and dividing numbers.

Normally you would have about two hours for a test like this, but for now, don't worry about timing. Just take the test in as relaxed a manner as you can. The answer sheet you should use for answering the questions is on the following page. Then comes the exam itself, and after that is the answer key, with each correct answer explained. The answer key is followed by a section on how to score your exam.

1. ⓐ ⓑ ⓒ ⓓ
2. ⓐ ⓑ ⓒ ⓓ
3. ⓐ ⓑ ⓒ ⓓ
4. ⓐ ⓑ ⓒ ⓓ
5. ⓐ ⓑ ⓒ ⓓ
6. ⓐ ⓑ ⓒ ⓓ
7. ⓐ ⓑ ⓒ ⓓ
8. ⓐ ⓑ ⓒ ⓓ
9. ⓐ ⓑ ⓒ ⓓ
10. ⓐ ⓑ ⓒ ⓓ
11. ⓐ ⓑ ⓒ ⓓ
12. ⓐ ⓑ ⓒ ⓓ
13. ⓐ ⓑ ⓒ ⓓ
14. ⓐ ⓑ ⓒ ⓓ
15. ⓐ ⓑ ⓒ ⓓ
16. ⓐ ⓑ ⓒ ⓓ
17. ⓐ ⓑ ⓒ ⓓ
18. ⓐ ⓑ ⓒ ⓓ
19. ⓐ ⓑ ⓒ ⓓ
20. ⓐ ⓑ ⓒ ⓓ
21. ⓐ ⓑ ⓒ ⓓ
22. ⓐ ⓑ ⓒ ⓓ
23. ⓐ ⓑ ⓒ ⓓ
24. ⓐ ⓑ ⓒ ⓓ

25. ⓐ ⓑ ⓒ ⓓ
26. ⓐ ⓑ ⓒ ⓓ
27. ⓐ ⓑ ⓒ ⓓ
28. ⓐ ⓑ ⓒ ⓓ
29. ⓐ ⓑ ⓒ ⓓ
30. ⓐ ⓑ ⓒ ⓓ
31. ⓐ ⓑ ⓒ ⓓ
32. ⓐ ⓑ ⓒ ⓓ
33. ⓐ ⓑ ⓒ ⓓ
34. ⓐ ⓑ ⓒ ⓓ
35. ⓐ ⓑ ⓒ ⓓ
36. ⓐ ⓑ ⓒ ⓓ
37. ⓐ ⓑ ⓒ ⓓ
38. ⓐ ⓑ ⓒ ⓓ
39. ⓐ ⓑ ⓒ ⓓ
40. ⓐ ⓑ ⓒ ⓓ
41. ⓐ ⓑ ⓒ ⓓ
42. ⓐ ⓑ ⓒ ⓓ
43. ⓐ ⓑ ⓒ ⓓ
44. ⓐ ⓑ ⓒ ⓓ
45. ⓐ ⓑ ⓒ ⓓ
46. ⓐ ⓑ ⓒ ⓓ
47. ⓐ ⓑ ⓒ ⓓ
48. ⓐ ⓑ ⓒ ⓓ

49. ⓐ ⓑ ⓒ ⓓ
50. ⓐ ⓑ ⓒ ⓓ
51. ⓐ ⓑ ⓒ ⓓ
52. ⓐ ⓑ ⓒ ⓓ
53. ⓐ ⓑ ⓒ ⓓ
54. ⓐ ⓑ ⓒ ⓓ
55. ⓐ ⓑ ⓒ ⓓ
56. ⓐ ⓑ ⓒ ⓓ
57. ⓐ ⓑ ⓒ ⓓ
58. ⓐ ⓑ ⓒ ⓓ
59. ⓐ ⓑ ⓒ ⓓ
60. ⓐ ⓑ ⓒ ⓓ
61. ⓐ ⓑ ⓒ ⓓ
62. ⓐ ⓑ ⓒ ⓓ
63. ⓐ ⓑ ⓒ ⓓ
64. ⓐ ⓑ ⓒ ⓓ
65. ⓐ ⓑ ⓒ ⓓ
66. ⓐ ⓑ ⓒ ⓓ
67. ⓐ ⓑ ⓒ ⓓ
68. ⓐ ⓑ ⓒ ⓓ
69. ⓐ ⓑ ⓒ ⓓ
70. ⓐ ⓑ ⓒ ⓓ

SANITATION WORKER EXAM 1

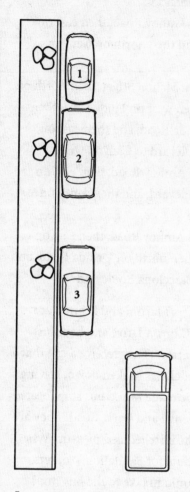

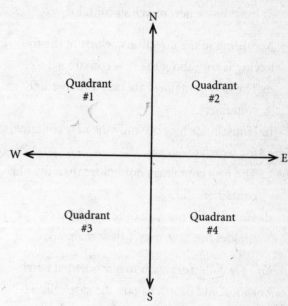

1. In the street scene shown above, which would be the best place for the driver to position the collection truck so that workers can load all three piles of garbage without moving the truck or touching any of the cars?
   a. in front of car 1
   b. between cars 1 and 2
   c. between cars 2 and 3
   d. behind car 3

2. Jean is standing at the intersection of the two lines shown above. If she travels north for two blocks, then west for three blocks, then south for four blocks, and then east for five blocks, in which quadrant will she end up?
   a. Quadrant #1
   b. Quadrant #2
   c. Quadrant #3
   d. Quadrant #4

Answer questions 3 and 4 on the basis of the following information.

The city has distributed standardized recycling containers to all households, with directions that read: "We would prefer that you use this new container as your primary recycling container. Additional recycling containers may be purchased from the city."

3. According to the directions, each household
   a. may only use one recycling container
   b. must use the new recycling container
   c. should use the new recycling container
   d. must buy a new recycling container

4. According to the directions, which of the following is true about the new containers?
   a. The new containers are better than other containers.
   b. Households may use only the new containers for recyclable items.
   c. The new containers hold more than the old containers did.
   d. Households may use other containers besides the new ones if they wish.

5. You are collecting trash in a residential neighborhood and drop a bag on the sidewalk. The bag splits, and four items fall out: a plastic coat hanger, a razor blade, a closed pocket knife, and a soldering iron. Which item is the most dangerous one for you to handle?
   a. plastic coat hanger
   b. razor blade
   c. closed pocket knife
   d. soldering iron

Answer questions 6–8 solely on the basis of the map on the facing page. The arrows indicate traffic flow; one arrow indicates a one-way street going in the direction of the arrow; two arrows represent a two-way street. You are not allowed to go the wrong way on a one-way street.

6. Sanitation Workers Kazinski and Benning are completing a routine pick-up at the Livingston Avenue Mall at the southeast corner of the building. Dispatch notifies them of a special

pick-up at a residence located at the northwest corner of Canyon Drive and Linda Lane. What is the quickest route for Kazinski and Benning to take to the residence?
   a. turn north on Amhoy Road, then east on Linda Lane, and then north on Canyon Drive
   b. turn east on McMahon Street, then north on El Camino, then west on Linda Lane, then north on Orinda Road, and then east on Barcelona Boulevard to Canyon Drive
   c. turn north on Amhoy Road, then east on Barcelona Boulevard, and then south on Canyon Drive
   d. turn north on Amhoy Road, then east on Bortz Road, then north on Orinda Road, and then east on Barcelona Boulevard

7. Sanitation Workers Martini and Schmid are southbound on Canyon Drive and have just crossed Edward Street. They receive a call that a city collection truck has broken down, leaving one pick-up to be made near a bus stop located at Livingston Avenue and Bortz Road. They are asked to make the unscheduled pick-up. What is the quickest route for Sanitation Workers Martini and Schmid to take to the bus stop?
   a. continue south on Canyon Drive, then west on McMahon Street, then north on Orinda Road, then west on Edward Street, then north on Amhoy Road, and then west on Bortz Road to Livingston Avenue
   b. continue south on Canyon Drive, then west on Lake Drive, and then north on Livingston Avenue to Bortz Road
   c. make a U-turn on Canyon Drive, and then go west on Bortz Road to Livingston Avenue

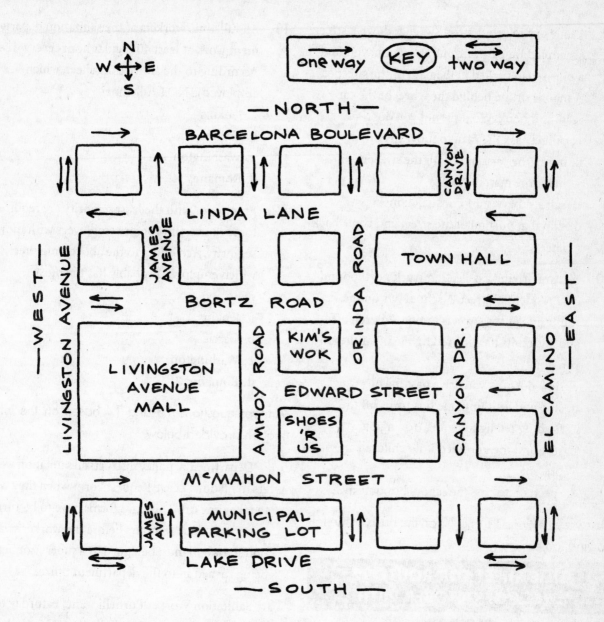

d. continue south on Canyon Drive, then east on Lake Drive, then north on El Camino, and then west on Bortz Road to Livingston Avenue

8. Sanitation Shift Supervisor Richfield is driving west on Bortz Road. She makes a right onto James Avenue, then a left onto Linda Lane, then a right onto Livingston Avenue, and then a right onto Barcelona Boulevard. What direction is she facing?

a. east

b. south

c. west

d. north

9. While driving your street sweeper down a street scheduled for cleaning one afternoon, you find a blue sedan parked in the path of the sweeper. A man is sitting behind the wheel of the car reading a book. What should you do?
   a. politely ask the man to move his car
   b. bump the car gently with the sweeper to make the man move
   c. call a supervisor for instructions
   d. skip that portion of the street and come back later

10. You are driving a collection truck northbound on a residential street. A school bus on the south side of the street is letting children off and has on its flashing red lights. What should you do?
    a. slow down as you drive past the bus
    b. stop and wait until the bus turns off the flashing red lights before driving on
    c. stop and then proceed if no children are present
    d. speed up to pass the school bus quickly

Answer questions 11 and 12 on the basis of the following table.

TIME SHEET FOR ROUTE 92, WEEK OF OCTOBER 20TH

WORKER	REGULAR HOURS	OVERTIME
Jenkins	40	2
Garcia	38	1
Washington	40	0
Romanov	40	5

11. All full-time workers at the sanitation department work at least 40 regular hours every week. According to the above time sheet, which employee is NOT full-time?
    a. Jenkins
    b. Garcia
    c. Washington
    d. Romanov

12. Employees with the least seniority are required to work overtime before employees with more seniority. According to the above time sheet, which employee probably has the most seniority?
    a. Jenkins
    b. Garcia
    c. Washington
    d. Romanov

Answer questions 13 and 14 based on the information provided below.

Departmental policy instructs all sanitation workers to fill out a Leave Request Form when they want to take time off. The leave forms have to be turned in no later than 48 hours before the worker's vacation starts and must be signed by a supervisor before being turned in to the department office.

13. Sanitation Worker Purnelli wants Saturday off to take his son to a baseball game. He asks his supervisor on Wednesday and is told to fill out a Leave Request Form. After he fills out the form, he should
    a. turn it in to the department office immediately
    b. wait until Friday afternoon to turn it in
    c. make sure the supervisor signs the form
    d. have a coworker who can cover for him on Saturday sign the form

14. To make sure she gets days off that she wants, Sanitation Worker Chow turns in her leave form one month ahead of time. The front office returns the form to her a few days later because she forgot to have her supervisor sign the form. What should she do now?
   a. cancel her vacation because it's too late to turn the new paperwork in
   b. fill out a new form and have her supervisor sign it
   c. have her supervisor sign the form and then turn it in again
   d. fill out a new form and submit it 48 hours before her vacation

15. You've just come from a meeting where employees were told to report on-the-job injuries to the supervisor as soon as they happen. As you hook up a snow plow to a truck, you cut your right thumb. The cut is fairly deep but only hurts a little. What should you do?
   a. put a bandage on your thumb and report the injury after you finish your task
   b. tell the supervisor about the injury after the end of the shift
   c. wait and see if the injury needs medical attention before you tell your supervisor
   d. report the injury immediately

16. A city ordinance reads "Residential garbage is defined as that produced by households in single-family dwellings or buildings with no more than two residential units." This means that
   a. the garbage produced by a family-owned business is not residential garbage
   b. only residences produce refuse defined as "garbage"

   c. the garbage produced by multi-unit apartment buildings is residential garbage
   d. only residential garbage will be picked up by the city

17. If a street sweeper travels at the speed of 15 mph for 2.5 hours, how far will it travel? (Distance = Rate × Time)
   a. 3.75 miles
   b. 10.5 miles
   c. 17.5 miles
   d. 37.5 miles

Answer questions 18 and 19 on the basis of the following information.

After a snow or ice fall, the city streets are treated with ordinary rock salt. In some areas, the salt is combined with calcium chloride, which is more effective in below-zero temperatures and better melts ice. This combination of salt and calcium chloride is also less damaging to foliage along the roadways.

18. In deciding whether to use ordinary rock salt or the salt and calcium chloride on a particular street, which of the following is NOT a consideration?
   a. the temperature at the time of treatment
   b. the plants and trees along the street
   c. whether there is ice on the street
   d. whether the street is a main or secondary road

19. According to the snow treatment directions, which of the following is true?
   a. If the temperature is below zero, salt and calcium chloride is effective in treating snow- and ice-covered streets.
   b. Crews must wait until the snow or ice stops falling before salting streets.
   c. The city always salts major roads first.
   d. If the snow fall is light, the city will not salt the streets as this would be a waste of the salt supply.

Answer questions 20 and 21 on the basis of the following information.

Only supervisors of the sanitation department are qualified to handle hazardous waste. Hazardous waste is defined as any waste designated hazardous by the United States Environmental Protection Agency. If a sanitation worker is unclear as to whether a particular item is hazardous, he or she should not handle the item but instead should notify the supervisor for directions.

20. Sanitation Worker Wong comes upon a container of cleaning solvent that has been set out along with the regular garbage in front of a residence. The container does not list the contents of the cleaner. Wong should
   a. contact the supervisor for directions
   b. assume the solvent is safe and deposit it in the sanitation truck
   c. leave a note for the residents asking them to list the contents of the container
   d. leave the container on the curb

21. On the basis of the passage, which of the following is the best definition of hazardous waste?
   a. anything that would be life-threatening to sanitation workers
   b. anything picked up by special sanitation trucks
   c. anything so defined by the United States Environmental Protection Agency
   d. anything not allowed with regular residential garbage

22. The cost of a list of supplies for a sanitation crew is as follows: $19.98, $52.20, $12.64, and $7.79. What is the total cost?
   a. $91.30
   b. $92.61
   c. $93.60
   d. $93.61

23. District 5 of one city's sanitation department serves about 21,500 residents. Of these, 11,350 live in single-family dwellings. About what percent of the district's residents live in single-family dwellings?
   a. 47%
   b. 49%
   c. 51%
   d. 53%

Answer questions 24–26 based on the following procedure.

Sanitation Department procedure for drivers who check out vehicles state that all sanitation vehicles are to be inspected for damage and to see if they operate properly before being driven on the road. The driver of each vehicle is responsible for walking around his or her vehicle and checking for the following situations:

1. puddles of fluid underneath the vehicle indicating a leak

2. burnt out tail lights, turn signals, hazard lights, or headlights

3. damage such as dents or paint damage

4. low tire pressure and loose lug nuts

24. Sanitation Worker Tsun has a meeting with his supervisor one morning which makes him a little late starting his route. He jogs to his collection truck, eager to get on the road. At this point, Tsun should

a. skip the inspection just this once to make up for lost time

b. check only the tires because they are the most important safety feature

c. check only for problems that make the vehicle unsafe to drive

d. inspect the vehicle fully even though it will make him later for his run

25. Sanitation Worker Rodriquez checks out one truck and performs the inspection. The truck engine won't start so he turns this truck back in for repair and checks out another truck. He should

a. perform the complete vehicle inspection on the new truck

b. skip the vehicle inspection because he's already done one this morning

c. check to make sure that the engine starts and then begin his route

d. look for puddles of fluid and then check all lights and the tires

26. Sanitation Worker Luhan and Sanitation Worker Ratchet will be riding together today. Luhan is the driver so she checks out the vehicle. What should she do next?

a. check the lights and look under the vehicle while Ratchet checks the body and tires

b. call a mechanic to do the inspection so she'll be sure it's done right

c. start the truck while Ratchet performs the inspection

d. check under the vehicle, and then check the lights, the body, and the tires

Answer questions 27–29 on the basis of the following graph.

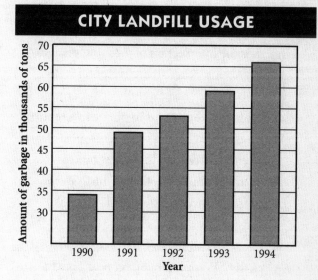

CITY LANDFILL USAGE

27. How many tons of garbage were deposited in the landfill in 1992?

a. 53

b. 530

c. 5,300

d. 53,000

28. Which period had the greatest increase in garbage?

a. 1990–1991

b. 1991–1992

c. 1992–1993

d. 1993–1994

29. If the trend indicated by the chart continues, what can the city expect about the amount of garbage deposited in the landfill in 1995?

a. The amount will be less than in 1994.

b. The amount will be more than in 1994.

c. The amount will be the same as in 1994.

d. The amount will be twice as much as in 1994.

30. An hour after a wind storm, Sanitation Worker Garcia is driving north on Washington Street when he comes upon a large tree limb that has fallen and is blocking his lane. About fifty yards north is the intersection of Washington and Fourth Avenue where there is a public telephone booth. Garcia carefully drives around the fallen limb and stops to phone in a report. Which of the following statements most clearly and accurately reports this situation?

a. I'm at the phone booth on Fourth Avenue in my truck, and a tree limb fell, which is blocking my lane.

b. A large tree limb has fallen across the road north of Washington Street near Fourth Avenue.

c. There is a fallen tree limb blocking one lane of Washington Street, about fifty yards south of Fourth Avenue.

d. In the northbound lane of Fourth Avenue and Washington Street, I had to drive around a limb that fell off a tree obstructing traffic.

31. A street sign affixed below a stop sign reads "Opposing traffic does not stop." What is the meaning of the sign?

a. A driver intending to turn right does not need to stop.

b. A driver approaching the sign needs only to slow down and proceed cautiously.

c. Vehicles coming directly toward the driver do not have a stop sign.

d. Vehicles approaching this sign must stop and wait for cross traffic to pass.

Answer questions 32–34 by choosing the word or phrase that means the same or nearly the same as the underlined word.

32. Shift supervisor Riggs gave a <u>plausible</u> explanation for being late for work.

a. incredible

b. insufficient

c. apologetic

d. believable

33. The corporation's habit of placing toxic materials in unmarked containers <u>aroused</u> anger in many sanitation workers.

a. informed

b. disappointed

c. provoked

d. deceived

34. Regarding the need stricter guidelines for garbage containers, the City Council's vote was <u>unanimous</u>.

a. divided

b. uniform

c. adamant

d. secure

Answer questions 35 and 36 on the basis of the following information.

The city ordinance reads, "Sanitation workers will not collect garbage in containers weighing more than fifty pounds." Workers are expected to use their best judgment in determining when a container weighs more than fifty pounds. If a container is too heavy, workers should attach one of the pre-printed warning messages (which are carried in all trucks) to the container, informing the household that the container weighs more than fifty pounds and cannot be collected.

35. According to the passage, in order to determine if a container is too heavy, sanitation workers should
   a. carry a scale in their truck to weigh containers
   b. practice lifting fifty pounds at home to know what it feels like
   c. assume any container he or she can lift weighs less than fifty pounds
   d. use her or his best guess as to whether a container weighs more than fifty pounds

36. According to the passage, if a sanitation worker believes that a container weighs more than fifty pounds, he or she should
   a. attach a warning to the container and leave it where it is
   b. leave it, but write a note to the household informing them of the weight limit
   c. collect it one time, but leave a note for the household explaining the weight limit
   d. notify a special collections truck to pick up the item

37. You and your partner are collecting garbage in front of Sandstone Apartments. You try to pick up a large box but have to strain because it is very heavy. What should you do?
   a. ask your partner for help
   b. leave the box on the sidewalk
   c. drag the box to the truck
   d. squat and lift from your legs

38. An angry citizen walks up to you and tells you that she wants to make a formal complaint about the collection service. What should you do?
   a. write down the woman's complaint and hand it to your supervisor at the end of your shift
   b. refer the woman to the proper office for handling customer complaints
   c. explain that you have no control over collection service policy and keep working
   d. promise the woman that the department will investigate and, if the complains are justified, will make the changes she wants

Answer questions 39 and 40 by choosing the word or phrase that means the same or nearly the same as the underlined word.

39. The collection trucks used by sanitation departments in the surrounding small towns are definitely <u>outmoded</u>.
   a. worthless
   b. unusable
   c. obsolete
   d. unnecessary

40. The new ruling regarding disposal of hypodermic needles may prove <u>detrimental</u> to the health of sanitation workers.
   a. decisive
   b. harmful
   c. worthless
   d. advantageous

41. You pick up a trash container at 215 Mocking-bird Lane and find a wallet in the container. The wallet has a twenty-dollar bill inside, along with a driver's license for a 70-year-old man named John Smith at 215 Mockingbird Lane. A man about that age, who resembles the picture on the driver's license, is sitting on the porch at this address. What should you do?

a. ask the man if he is John Smith and, if so, give him back the wallet

b. assume the wallet was discarded deliberately and keep it

c. turn the wallet in to your supervisor at the end of your shift

d. leave the wallet in the trash

42. Sanitation Worker Davis is driving east on First Avenue when a large dog runs in front of his truck. Davis slams on his brakes but is unable to keep from hitting the dog. Hearing the screeching of the brakes, the dog's owner, James Ramsey, runs out of his house on the corner of First Avenue and Highland Court and discovers that his dog's leg is injured. Davis helps put the dog into Ramsey's car so that Ramsey can take the animal to the vet. Later, Davis files a report. Which of the following reports describes the incident most clearly and accurately?

a. The dog's owner, James Ramsey, whose leg appeared to be broken, took him to the vet after I helped him into the car on First Avenue at Highland Court.

b. Near the intersection of First Avenue and Highland Court, a dog ran out in front of my truck and I could not avoid hitting it. I stopped to help the dog's owner, James Ramsey, who took the injured animal to the vet.

c. I was driving along First Avenue when I hit a dog. We picked the dog up with a leg injury and put him in the car, which then drove to the vet. James Ramsey was the man's name.

d. James Ramsey, who owned a dog, came running out of his house at First and Highland and saw me hit him with my truck. Though I didn't mean to do it, I helped him into a car so that Ramsey could get to the vet for medical treatment.

43. Sanitation Worker Roth is loading a collection truck with trash in the alley behind the apartment building at 4498 Cahill Avenue when she hears someone calling for help. She looks up and sees an older man at the window on the third floor. The man shouts that his wife may have had a heart attack and his phone is out of order. Roth goes into the building and calls 911 from the superintendent's phone. Which of the following statements reports the emergency most clearly and accurately?

a. Send an ambulance to the apartment building at 4498 Cahill Avenue. A woman on the third floor may have had a heart attack.

b. In the alley behind 4498 Cahill Avenue, a woman may have suffered a heart attack and needs an ambulance.

c. The woman's husband on the third floor of the apartment building said she had a heart attack, but his phone is out of order.

d. An ambulance is immediately needed at 4498 Cahill Avenue. I spoke to the victim's husband in the alley behind the building where she had a heart attack.

44. Sanitation Worker Camillo is stopped for a red light on Lucas Drive. When the light turns green, Camillo drives slowly forward into the intersection of Lucas Drive and Manchester Way. There, his truck is broadsided from the left by a gray, late-model Mercury station wagon. Although he is shaken, Camillo has not been injured. The driver of the car is also uninjured, but he accuses Camillo of having driven through a red light. Someone in a nearby building saw the accident and phoned the police, who arrive within minutes. Which of the following reports would Camillo give to the police to describe the accident most clearly and accurately?

a. I was on Lucas, completely stopped for the red light. Then, when the light turned green, I pulled forward and was immediately broadsided by the gray Mercury station wagon.

b. He's accusing me of going through a red light, but before I drove through I stopped. I didn't see the station wagon as it hit the left side of the truck coming down Manchester Way.

c. The station wagon drove into the side of my truck when I tried to drive forward on Lucas Drive. It was after the red light. Then he accused me of causing the accident.

d. I was driving straight ahead on Lucas Drive, and when I was at the light at the intersection of Manchester Way, I pulled forward and he hit me. It was a gray Mercury station wagon.

45. On designated holidays, there is no garbage collection in the city. When a holiday falls on a Monday, sanitation workers collect their normal Monday route and half of their normal Tuesday route on the Tuesday after the holiday. On the next day, Wednesday, they collect the second half of their normal Tuesday route and all of their normal Wednesday route. On Wednesday, September 6, two days after a holiday, the resident at 456 Dornan Street phones the city's Sanitation Department to complain that his garbage, which is normally collected on Tuesdays, is still sitting in front of his house. Which of the following explanations would describe most clearly and accurately to this resident why his garbage has not yet been collected?

a. Because your route is usually on Tuesday, your garbage will now be collected on Wednesday when there is a holiday.

b. Don't worry. Your garbage will be picked up sometime today because half the route you are on was picked up yesterday, and you're on the second half.

c. When there is a holiday on Monday, as there was this week, your garbage will be collected on Wednesday.

d. Because of Monday's holiday, the garbage could not be collected, which is why yours is still there. Some of the people whose garbage is collected on Tuesdays, however, did have their normal collection day.

46. One rainy afternoon you are picking up trash in a residential neighborhood. You have just gotten back into your truck to drive to the next pick-up point, when you see an elderly woman about half a block away, walking toward you, struggling to carry a small bag of trash. What should you do?

a. drive on, as regulations state all trash should be set out before pickup time

b. wait for the woman to bring the trash to you, but thank her for her efforts

c. drive on, as it is extremely important not to be late driving a pick-up route

d. get out of the truck, walk to the woman, and take the trash from her

47. When you stop your collection truck to pick up trash along a busy city street, a small boy grabs the side mirror on the driver's side and hangs there, shouting for you to take him for a ride. What should you do?

a. drive the boy slowly down the street a few feet and then ask him to get off

b. open the door quickly to dump him onto the sidewalk

c. don't move the truck and tell the boy to get down immediately

d. tell the boy you will call the police if you see him at that corner again

48. You are driving a sand spreader along an icy street. You are driving slowly, and when you step on the brakes to stop you realize they do not work. You ease the emergency brake on until the vehicle stops completely. What should you do now?

a. keep sanding the street and use the emergency brake in place of the regular brakes

b. do not drive the vehicle any further and call the situation in to the supervisor

c. drive the vehicle directly back to the maintenance yard

d. wait where you are until police or a city tow truck comes along

Answer questions 49–51 solely on the basis of the map on the facing page. The arrows indicate traffic flow; one arrow indicates a one-way street going in the direction of the arrow; two arrows represent a two-way street. You are not allowed to go the wrong way on a one-way street.

49. Sanitation Worker Tennyson is eastbound on Kent Avenue at Lee Lane. He receives a call about assistance needed for a pick-up at a residence located at the northeast corner of Lynch Road and Mill Road. What is the quickest route for Sanitation Worker Tennyson to take?

a. continue east on Kent Avenue, then north on Main Street to Mill Road, and then west on Mill Road to the northeast corner of Lynch Road and Mill Road

b. continue east on Kent Avenue, then north on Main Street, then west on Pomeroy Boulevard, and then south on Lynch Road

c. continue east on Kent Avenue, then south on Main Street, then west on Pine Avenue, then north on Grove Street, and then east on Mill Road to Lynch Road

d. continue east on Kent Avenue, then north on Main Street, then west on Palmer Avenue, and then north on Lynch Road to Mill Road

50. There has been heavy flooding in the city and, on an emergency basis, some collection routes are being canceled or reassigned. Sanitation Workers McKay and Callihan are driving by the court house, northbound on Upton Street. They receive a call that their regular route is being canceled, and that instead they are to

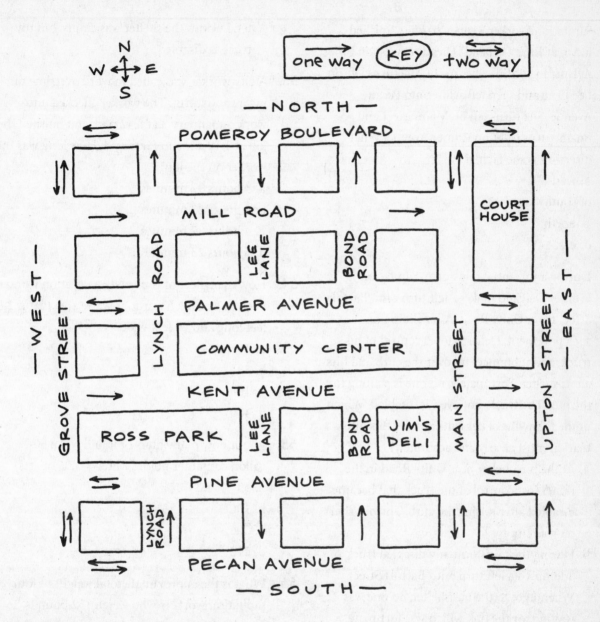

begin pick-up at Ross Park on the Grove Street side of the park. What is the most direct legal route for Sanitation Workers McKay and Callihan to take?

a. continue north on Upton Street, and then drive west on Pomeroy Boulevard, then south on Main Street, and then west on Kent Avenue to Grove Street

b. continue north on Upton Street, and then drive then west on Pomeroy Boulevard, and then south on Grove Street to Ross Park

c. continue north on Upton Street, and then drive west on Pomeroy Boulevard, then south on Main Street, then west on Pecan Avenue, and then north on Grove Street to Ross Park

d. make a U-turn on Upton Street and then go west on Palmer Avenue and then south on Grove Street to Ross Park

51. Sanitation Worker Kenney has just finished lunch at Jim's Deli and is heading west on Pine Avenue to continue her route. She turns left on Lee Lane and then left again onto Pecan Avenue. She turns left on Main Street and finally turns right on Palmer Avenue. What direction is she facing?

a. west
b. south
c. north
d. east

52. During a torrential rainstorm, Sanitation Worker Delgado makes a left turn onto Bartola Street from Unity Road. After sliding on the slick pavement, Delgado loses control of his truck, and it bounces up over the curb and hits a bus shelter. Fortunately, no one is waiting for the bus. The truck, however, is disabled. Which of the following statements reports this information most clearly and accurately?

a. At the bus shelter near Unity Road in the rain, I lost control of the truck that became disabled after hitting the curb. The bus shelter was empty.

b. During the rainstorm, my disabled truck attempted a left turn onto Bartola Street. When I got to the bus shelter, no one was waiting for the bus, which was fortunate when I lost control and ran up over the curb.

c. From Unity Road, I missed the turn onto Bartola Street after I lost control of the truck. It bounced over the curb, which hit the bus shelter. Although the truck is disabled, the shelter did not sustain any injuries.

d. As I was turning left onto Bartola Street from Unity Road, the truck slid on the wet pavement. I lost control and hit the bus shel-

ter. Luckily, the shelter was empty, but my truck is disabled.

53. A city worker was called to work overtime during a snowstorm. The worker checked into work on January 3 at 8:42 p.m. and finished the job at 1:19 a.m. on January 4. How long was the worker on the job?

a. 3 hours 37 minutes
b. 4 hours 23 minutes
c. 4 hours 37 minutes
d. 5 hours 23 minutes

54. How many feet of rope will a sanitation worker need to tie off a hazardous waste area that is 34 feet long and 20 feet wide?

a. 56
b. 88
c. 108
d. 480

55. About how many liters of liquid will a 50-gallon container hold? (1 liter = 1.06 quarts)

a. 53
b. 106
c. 206
d. 212

56. What is the approximate total weight of four sanitation workers who weigh 152 pounds, 168 pounds, 182 pounds, and 201 pounds?

a. 690 pounds
b. 700 pounds
c. 710 pounds
d. 750 pounds

57. If a compartment on the back of a recycling truck is 10 feet long, 6 feet wide, and 4 feet high, what is its volume in cubic feet? (Volume = Length × Width × Height)

a. 20

b. 64

c. 210

d. 240

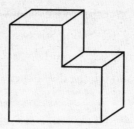

58. One morning you are carrying an old sofa to the truck with the help of your coworker, when your coworker trips, falls, and hits her head on the sidewalk. She is unconscious. What should you do?

a. use the truck radio to call for help

b. shake her until she wakes up

c. pick her up and place her on the sofa

d. hold up her head and give her some water

59. You are behind schedule sweeping up trash near a busy downtown intersection. A tourist stops and asks you if you know how to get to Wilson's Pie Shop. You know that this shop is in a mall at least a mile away, and that giving directions would be time-consuming. What should you do?

a. advise the tourist to find a city map

b. tell the tourist you are late getting your work done and therefore can't answer

c. give the tourist directions to the store

d. call a supervisor over to deal with the unwelcome interruption

60. Which of the following figures could be the object above, seen from a different angle?

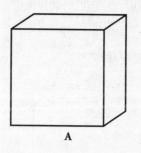

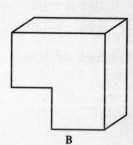

A   B

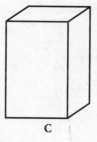

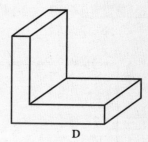

C   D

a. B only

b. A and B

c. B and C

d. B and D

61. While driving a sweeper, you see smoke billowing out of a window at 3939 Walking Stick Lane. What is the first thing you should do?

a. call in on your radio and tell the dispatcher to call for a fire truck

b. stop a passerby and ask that person to call 911

c. drive to the next street because fire trucks will need to drive down this street

d. stop your truck and approach the building to see if you can help anyone inside

Question 62 refers to the figures below.

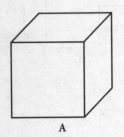

A

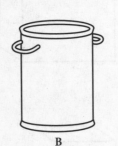

B

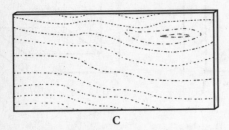

C

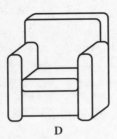

D

62. If each of the objects to the left weighs approximately 40 pounds, which would be easiest for one sanitation worker alone to carry to the collection truck?

a. Object A

b. Object B

c. Object C

d. Object D

63. While Sanitation Worker Yamata is making a garbage pickup at an apartment building in the 700 block of Norcross Road, two boys run up to his truck and spray graffiti on the driver's side door. Yamata, who is busy with the collection, does not see the boys. Mrs. Stanley, who is walking her dog, is the only witness to the crime. She stops Yamata and tells him that one of the boys, Randy McGill, age thirteen, lives in the 800 block of Norcross. When Yamata returns to the garage, he files a report. Which of the following reports most clearly and accurately states what occurred?

a. On the 700 block of Norcross Road, which I was picking up, Mrs. Stanley told me about the graffiti on the truck. It appeared there after teenagers living on the next block ran down Norcross with a spray can. It was on the driver's side.

b. Mrs. Stanley was walking her dog and said that Randy McGill lived in the next block of Norcross from the one I was doing the pickup. He was thirteen and spray painted the truck, but I did not get an eyewitness myself because I was busy with the pickup.

c. Mrs. Stanley and her dog told me that Randy McGill lived in the 800 block of Norcross while I was making my pickup in the 700 block. He was thirteen with another boy, and

I was told that they were the ones to spray the graffiti. However, I did not witness this myself.

d. As I was making a pickup in the 700 block of Norcross Road, Mrs. Stanley witnessed two boys spraying graffiti on the driver's side of my truck. She identified one of the boys as thirteen-year-old Randy McGill who lives in the 800 block of Norcross.

64. Sanitation Worker Green earns $26,000 a year. If she receives a 4.5% salary increase, how much will she earn?
a. $26,450
b. $27,170
c. $27,260
d. $29,200

65. Which of the following areas has the greatest perimeter?
a. a square 11 feet by 11 feet
b. a square 10 feet by 10 feet
c. a rectangle 12 feet by 8 feet
d. a rectangle 14 feet by 7 feet

66. It's raining heavily and you can't see the street in front of the collection truck even with the windshield wipers on their fastest setting. What should you do?
a. pull over as soon as possible and wait until the rain lets up a bit before driving on
b. drive back to the maintenance yard and ask them to put on better windshield wipers
c. roll down the window and hang your head out to see better
d. keep driving very slowly

67. The city's new collection program will begin June 1. At that time, each house or apartment will be allowed two 35-gallon cans or bags of garbage per week. Each additional bag or can will require a special sticker. Stickers may be purchased from the city at $1.00 each. Which of the following statements describes the city's new program most clearly and accurately?
a. On June 1, 35-gallon cans or bags must have a sticker on them that can be purchased from the city for $1.00. Each resident will be allowed two cans or bags.
b. Beginning June 1, the city will limit each household to two 35-gallon cans or bags. Additional cans or bags must carry stickers, which can be purchased from the city for $1.00 each.
c. With the city's new collection program, each person will be able to have two cans or bags of garbage. After June 1, stickers must be purchased for additions, which cost $1.00 per can or bag.
d. Each week, each household will be required to have two 35-gallon bags or cans of garbage. Stickers will be placed, at $1.00 each purchased from the city, on additional cans or bags.

68. During a major snowstorm, Sanitation Worker O'Neal is driving a truck with a "quick hitch" plow along the 1200 block of Arden Drive, one of the city's main snow routes. When the snow is over two inches deep, residents are restricted from parking on streets that are designated snow routes. The snow on this day is already four inches deep. Suddenly, O'Neal sees a parked car on the left side of the street and barely manages to drive the truck around it. At the first opportunity, she phones in a request to have the car towed. Which of the following statements most clearly and accurately describes the situation?

a. Because I almost did not see the car on Arden Drive during this snowstorm, it should be removed immediately.

b. I am calling for a tow truck in the 1200 block of a main snow route, because I almost hit a car with the snow falling, which made it impossible to see cars on my left side.

c. As I was plowing the 1200 block of Arden Drive, I almost ran into an illegally parked car. Please send a tow truck and have the car removed.

d. There is a car in the 1200 block of Arden Drive. The snow is four inches deep, which may cause an accident and should be towed immediately.

69. At certain times of day, drivers of collection trucks should be particularly careful to look for pedestrians before starting up again after a collection stop. Drivers should look most carefully for pedestrians in the street at

a. 6:45 a.m. in a commercial district

b. 8:15 a.m. in a school zone

c. 10:30 a.m. in a residential neighborhood

d. 4:30 p.m. in an industrial park

70. City recycling regulations state that recyclable materials must be sorted and packaged separately for collection. If a householder does not follow these rules, sanitation workers are instructed not to do the pickup, but to leave a polite note. When Sanitation Worker Calhoun arrives at 29 Reynolds Lane, she discovers that newspaper, cans, glass jars, and plastic bottles have all been mingled together in one package. Which of the following notes would most clearly and accurately describe the situation to the resident at 29 Reynolds Lane?

a. When recycling, I did not pick up your materials because of the city recycling rules, which I was instructed not to do so.

b. I am sorry that I was unable to collect your recyclables today. City regulations require that recyclable materials be sorted and packaged separately.

c. The regulations of the city mean that I cannot pick up at 29 Reynolds Road when you aren't ready for collection. I am sorry about this inconvenience.

d. When recycling, I will not be able to pick up at this residence. Please note that city regulations require a pick up when materials are not left unsorted and in separate packages.

ANSWERS

1. c. There is enough space between cars 2 and 3 for workers to move the garbage without touching the cars. This position is closest to all three piles of garbage. Positioning the truck in front of car 1 or behind car 3 would require the workers to carry the garbage farther than necessary.

2. d. Jean travels two blocks farther to the south than she does to the north and two blocks farther to the east than she does to the west. Therefore, she finishes to the southeast of where she began, in Quadrant #4.

3. c. The directions indicate that the city prefers, but does not require, use of the new container provided by the city, and that the customers may use more than one container if they purchase an additional one.

4. d. The directions state the city would like households to use the new containers as their primary containers; this indicates that other containers are allowed.

5. b. A razor blade is a very sharp object and is far more likely to cause injury than any of the other choices.

6. c. This is the simplest way around the one-way streets and Town Hall. Because Linda Lane is one-way the wrong way, some backtracking is inevitable. However, the residence is only one block off of Barcelona Boulevard, and so turning east on Barcelona requires the least amount of backtracking. Choice **a** directs the sanitation workers to turn the wrong way down a one-way street. Choice **b** requires too much backtracking. Choice **d** leaves the workers on Barcelona Boulevard, not on Linda Lane.

7. b. This route is the most direct because it requires the fewest turns. Choice **a** requires the sanitation workers to go the wrong way on McMahon Street. Choice **c** is not correct because Canyon Drive is a one-way street south. Choice **d** takes the workers too far east.

8. a. If Shift Supervisor Richfield turns right onto James Avenue, she will be facing north. A left turn onto Linda Lane turns her west again, and a right turn onto Livingston Avenue turns her north. The final right turn onto Barcelona Boulevard turns her east.

9. a. It's quickest and most courteous to ask the man to move his car. Bumping the car (choice **b**) would be illegal. Not sweeping the street (choice **d**) would be irresponsible. Calling your supervisor (choice **c**) might be an option if the man refuses your request to move his vehicle.

10. b. The law requires all vehicles to come to a complete stop for school buses with flashing red lights.

11. b. Garcia is the only employee who worked less than 40 regular hours this week.

12. c. Washington is the only employee who did not work overtime; therefore, Washington probably has the most seniority.

13. c. The rule for requesting time off states that the form must be signed by a supervisor before it is turned in.

14. c. Although the office returned the form to Chow, the rule remains the same. She should get her supervisor to sign the form and then turn it back in, but there's no need for her to fill out a new form.

15. d. Ignoring a fairly deep cut would be unsafe. Also, ignoring a carefully defined work rule would be irresponsible.

16. a. The directions define residential garbage as *that produced by a household*, not by a business. Choices **b** and **d** are wrong, because they are not addressed in the definition. Choice **c** is clearly outside the scope of the definition.

17. d. Using the formula, this is a simple multiplication problem: 15 times 2.5 is 37.5.

18. d. The directions mention nothing about main or secondary roads.

19. a. The other choices are not mentioned in the directions.

20. a. The directions indicate that Wong should call the supervisor.

21. c. According to the passage, hazardous waste is *any waste designated hazardous by the United States Environmental Protection Agency.* The other choices are not mentioned.

22. b. You simply add all the numbers together to solve this problem.

23. d. Division is used to arrive at a decimal, which can then be rounded to the nearest hundredth and converted to a percentage: 11,350 divided by 21,500 is 0.5279. Then, 0.5279 rounded to the nearest hundredth is 0.53, or 53%.

24. d. The fact that Tsun is running late should have no impact on whether or not he performs the inspection. The inspection is important to the safety of the public as well as to his own safety.

25. a. Rodriquez is required to inspect all vehicles that he checks out. His inspection of the first vehicle should have no impact on whether he inspects the replacement vehicle. Choice **d** would have been a good choice except that it omits checking the body.

26. d. The rule says that the driver is responsible for performing the inspection. Since Luhan is the driver, she should perform the entire inspection, not just part of it.

27. d. The table lists the amounts of garbage in thousands of tons.

28. a. From 1990 to 1991 the amount of garbage deposited at the landfill increased by 15,000 tons.

29. b. For each year on the chart, the amount of garbage deposited in the landfill has increased. If the trend continues, it will increase in 1995 as well.

30. c. Choice **a** is incorrect because it leaves out information; choices **b** and **d** give incorrect information.

31. c. "Opposing traffic" means traffic coming directly toward the driver facing the sign.

32. d. *Plausible* means *believable.*

33. c. To *arouse* is to *provoke.*

34. b. If the vote was *unanimous,* everyone voted in the same way, so the vote was *uniform.*

35. d. Although the other options are not precluded by the passage, the directions require only that workers make an educated guess as to the weight of the container.

36. a. According to the passage, the worker should attach a *pre-printed warning message* and leave the container. The other choices are not mentioned.

37. a. One of the main reasons for assigning partners to work together is so that they can help each other. Leaving the box (choice **b**) would be irresponsible, as long as you and your partner can lift it without straining. Choices **c** and **d** are likely to lead to unnecessary injury.

38. b. By explaining to the customer the best place to handle her complaint, you've acted professionally. Taking the complaint yourself (choice **a**) would be a less professional option, as the complaint may not be addressed if it isn't made through the proper channels. Choice **c** would be rude and damaging to public relations. Choice **d** entails a promise you cannot be certain will be kept.

39. c. *Outmoded* means *obsolete.*

40. b. *Detrimental* means *harmful.*

41. a. In this situation, the common sense solution is to return the wallet to its owner if that's who the man turns out to be. Keeping the wallet (choice **b**) would be dishonest, and leaving it in the trash (choice **d**) would be irresponsible once you know its value. Giving the wallet to your supervisor (choice **c**) would be correct only if the man on the porch turns out not to be John Smith.

42. b. Choice **a** is incorrect because it implies that James Ramsey broke his leg; choice **c** leaves out information; choice **d** is unclear.

43. a. Choice **b** is incorrect because it implies that the woman is in the alley; choices **c** and **d** leave out important information.

44. a. Choices **b**, **c**, and **d** are incorrect because they leave out information and distort what really happened.

45. c. Choice **a** is incorrect because it leaves out information; choices **b** and **d** are unclear.

46. d. It would be courteous and good for public relations to help the woman, especially since it will take very little time. The other choices would be unnecessarily rude.

47. c. The only safe choice is to tell the boy to get off the truck immediately. As harmless as choices **a** and **b** might seem, injury could result. Choice **d** is incorrect because the boy has a right to be at the corner, and calling the police, or even threatening to do so, would be unjustified.

48. b. Faulty brakes are very dangerous, so the only safe solution is not to drive the vehicle. Choice **a** would be an inappropriate use of the emergency brake. Choice **c** would entail driving the truck. Choice **d** is incorrect because it is the sanitation department's responsibility to take care of truck maintenance; also, waiting for the police or a tow truck would waste time.

49. d. This is the most direct route because it does not require any backtracking. Choice **a** is not correct because it would require Sanitation Worker Tennyson to go the wrong way on Mill Road. Choice **b** requires some backtracking and takes the worker the wrong way on Lynch Road. Choice **c** is not as direct because it requires the worker to move in the opposite direction from the call.

50. b. This is the fastest route, requiring the fewest turns. Choice **a** is not correct because Kent is a one-way street going east. Choice **c** requires too many turns and is not the most direct route. Choice **d** is not correct because Upton Street is one-way going north.

51. d. A left turn onto Lee Lane turns Sanitation Worker Kenney south. Another left turn onto Pecan Avenue turns her east. A left turn onto Main Street turns her north, and the final right turn onto Palmer turns her back east.

52. d. Choice **a** is inaccurate; choice **b** leaves out information; choice **c** is both inaccurate and unclear.

53. c. Subtraction and addition will solve this problem. From 8:42 to 12:42, four hours elapse. From 12:42 to 1:00, another 18 minutes go by (60 − 42 = 18). Then, from 1:00 to 1:19, another 19 minutes pass.

54. c. There are two sides 34 feet long and two sides 20 feet long. Using the formula $P = 2L + 2W$ will solve this problem. Therefore, you should multiply 34 times 2 and 20 times 2 and add the results: $68 + 40 = 108$.

55. d. The answer to this question lies in knowing that there are four quarts to a gallon. There are therefore 200 quarts in a 50-gallon container. Multiply 200 by 1.06 quarts per liter to get 212 liters.

56. b. Add all four weights for a total of 703. 703 rounded to the nearest ten is 700.

57. d. This is a multiplication problem using the formula given: 10 times 6 times 4 is 240.

58. a. The only safe option is to call for help. The other choices would entail moving your coworker in some way; this could be dangerous as you cannot know what kind of injury she has.

59. c. A simple, courteous response is best here. The other responses would be impolite and might damage public relations for your department.

60. a. Figure B is the object rotated 180 degrees. None of the other figures corresponds to the object shown.

61. a. It will take only seconds to report the fire by radio, and your action could save lives or property. Choices **b** and **c** would waste valuable time. Choice **d** would also waste time, might be dangerous, and could interfere with professional firefighters' efforts.

62. b. The handles make the trash barrel relatively easy for one person to carry.

63. d. Choice **a** is unclear and distorts the facts; choices **b** and **c** provide most of the information but are unclear.

64. b. There are three steps involved in solving this problem. First, convert 4.5% to a decimal: 0.045. Multiply that by $26,000 to find out how much the salary increases. Finally, add the result ($1,170) to the original salary of $26,000 to find out the new salary, $27,170.

65. a. First you have to determine the perimeters of all four areas. This is done by using the formula for a square (P = 4S), or for a rectangle (P = 2L + 2W), as follows: $4 \times 11 = 44$ for choice **a**; $4 \times 10 = 40$ for choice **b**; $(2 \times 12) + (2 \times 8) = 40$ for choice **c**; and $(2 \times 14) + (2 \times 7) = 42$ for choice **d**. Choice **a** is greatest.

66. a. Continuing to drive would be unsafe, as you cannot see. Pulling over and letting the rain die down a bit makes the most sense.

67. b. Choice **a** is incorrect because it implies that all bags and cans must have a sticker; choice **c** gives all the information but is less clear than choice **b**; choice **d** is inaccurate.

68. c. Choice **a** is incorrect because it leaves out important information; choices **b** and **d** are unclear.

69. b. Though there may be pedestrians present at the other times and places listed, there are likely to be a lot of children on the street and sidewalks at 8:15 a.m. near a school.

70. b. Choices **a** and **c** do not clearly state why the recyclables were not picked up; choice **d** is unclear.

SCORING

In order to figure your total score on this exam, first find the number of questions you got right. Questions you skipped or got wrong don't count; just add up how many questions you got right out of the 70 questions on this exam. Then, in order to see how that score compares with a passing score, you'll have to convert that score to a percentage. This will be good practice for the math skills you need on the exam: divide your total score by 0.7 to find out what percentage of the questions you got right. (All right, you can use a calculator. But just this once.) The table below will help you check your work by giving you percentage equivalents for some possible scores.

Number of questions right	Approximate percentage
70	100%
65	93%
60	86%
55	79%
50	71%
45	64%
40	57%
35	50%

In most cities you need a score of 70 percent on the actual Sanitation Worker exam in order to pass. A few municipalities may use your written exam score to determine your rank on the eligibility list. If your city is one of those, you want the highest score you can possibly achieve in order to improve your chances of being hired. In most cities, however, simply passing with a score of 70 is enough—other factors determine whether you get the job.

What's much more important than your total score, for now, is how you did on each of the kinds of question on the exam. You need to diagnose your strengths and weaknesses so that you can concentrate your efforts as you prepare for the exam. As you probably noticed, the various kinds of questions are all mixed up together on the exam. So take out your completed answer sheet and compare it to the table on the next page. Find out which kinds of questions you did well in and which kinds gave you more trouble. Then you can plan to spend more of your preparation time on the chapters of this book that correspond to the questions you found hardest and less time on the chapters in areas in which you did well.

Even if you got a perfect score on a particular kind of question, you'll probably want to at least glance through the relevant chapter. On the other hand, you should spend a lot of time with the chapters on the question types that gave you the most difficulty, particularly if your total score was under 70 percent. After you work through those chapters, take the second practice exam in Chapter 11 to see how much you've improved.

Question type	Question numbers	Chapter
Understanding written language	3, 4, 11, 12, 16, 18–21, 27–29, 31, 35, 36	6, "Reading Comprehension"
Communicating information	30, 32–34, 39, 40, 42–45, 52, 63, 67, 68, 70	7, "Verbal Expression"
Using spatial reasoning	1, 2, 6–8, 49–51, 60, 62	8, "Map Reading and Spatial Relations"
Using judgment and following rules	5, 9, 10, 13–15, 24–26, 37, 38, 41, 46–48, 58, 59, 61, 66, 69	9, "Good Judgment and Common Sense"
Math	17, 22, 23, 53–57, 64, 65	10, "Math"

C·H·A·P·T·E·R 6

READING COMPREHENSION

CHAPTER SUMMARY

Because reading is such a vital skill, most civil service exams include a reading comprehension section that tests your ability to understand what you read. The tips and exercises in this chapter will help you improve your comprehension of written passages as well as of tables, charts, and graphs, so that you can increase your score in this area.

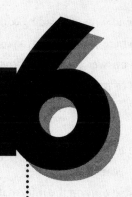 emos, policies, procedures, reports—these are all things you'll be expected to understand if you become a civil servant. Understanding written materials is part of almost any job. That's why most civil service tests attempt to measure how well applicants understand what they read.

Reading comprehension tests are usually in a multiple-choice format and ask questions based on brief passages, much like the standardized tests that are offered in schools. For that matter, almost all standardized test questions test your reading skill. After all, you can't answer the question if you can't read it! Similarly, you can't study your training materials or learn new procedures once you're on the job if you can't read well. So reading comprehension is vital not only on the test but also for the rest of your career.

TYPES OF READING COMPREHENSION QUESTIONS

You have probably encountered reading comprehension questions before, where you are given a passage to read and then have to answer multiple-choice questions about it. This kind of question has two advantages for you as a test taker:

1. You don't have to know anything about the topic of the passage because
2. You're being tested only on the information the passage provides.

But the disadvantage is that you have to know where and how to find that information quickly in an unfamiliar text. This makes it easy to fall for one of the wrong answer choices, especially since they're designed to mislead you.

The best way to do well on this passage/question format is to be very familiar with the kinds of questions that are typically asked on the test. Questions most frequently ask you to:

1. identify a specific **fact or detail** in the passage
2. note the **main idea** of the passage
3. make an **inference** based on the passage
4. define a **vocabulary** word from the passage

In order for you to do well on a reading comprehension test, you need to know exactly what each of these questions is asking. **Facts and details** are the specific pieces of information that support the passage's **main idea**. The main idea is the thought, opinion, or attitude that governs the whole passage. Generally speaking, facts and details are indisputable—things that don't need to be proven, like statistics (18 million people) or descriptions (a green overcoat). Let's say, for example, you read a sentence that says "*After the department's reorganization, workers were 50% more productive.*" A sentence like this, which gives you the **fact** that 50% of workers were more productive, might support a **main idea** that says, "*Every department should be reorganized.*" Notice that this main idea is not something indisputable; it is an opinion. The writer thinks all departments should be reorganized, and because this is his opinion (and not everyone shares it), he needs to support his opinion with facts and details.

An **inference**, on the other hand, is a conclusion that can be drawn based on fact or evidence. For example, you can infer—based on the fact that workers became 50% more productive after the reorganization, which is a dramatic change—that the department had not been efficiently organized. The fact sentence, "*After the department's reorganization, workers were 50% more productive,*" also implies that the reorganization of the department was the reason workers became more productive. There may, of course, have been other reasons, but we can infer only one from this sentence.

As you might expect, **vocabulary** questions ask you to determine the meaning of particular words. Often, if you've read carefully, you can determine the meaning of such words from their context, that is, how the word is used in the sentence or paragraph.

PRACTICE PASSAGE 1: USING THE FOUR QUESTION TYPES

The following is a sample test passage, followed by four questions. Read the passage carefully, and then answer the questions, based on your reading of the text, by circling your choice. Then refer to the list above and note under your answer which type of question has been asked. Correct answers appear immediately after the questions.

In the last decade, community policing has been frequently touted as the best way to reform urban law enforcement. The idea of putting more officers on foot patrol in high crime areas, where relations with police have frequently been strained, was initiated in Houston in 1983 under the leadership of then-Commissioner Lee Brown. He believed that officers should be accessible to the community at the street level. If officers were assigned to the same area over a period of time, those officers would eventually build a network of trust with neighborhood residents. That trust would mean that merchants and residents in the community would let officers know about criminal activities in the area and would support police intervention. Since then, many large cities have experimented with Community-Oriented Policing (COP) with mixed results. Some have found that police and citizens are grateful for the opportunity to work together. Others have found that unrealistic expectations by citizens and resistance from officers have combined to hinder the effectiveness of COP. It seems possible, therefore, that a good idea may need improvement before it can truly be considered a reform.

1. Community policing has been used in law enforcement since
   a. the late 1970s
   b. the early 1980s
   c. the Carter administration
   d. Lee Brown was New York City Police Commissioner

   Question type_____

2. The phrase "a network of trust" in this passage suggests that
   a. police officers can rely only on each other for support
   b. community members rely on the police to protect them
   c. police and community members rely on each other
   d. community members trust only each other

   Question type_____

3. The best title for this passage would be
   a. Community Policing: The Solution to the Drug Problem
   b. Houston Sets the Pace in Community Policing
   c. Communities and Cops: Partners for Peace
   d. Community Policing: An Uncertain Future?

   Question type_____

4. The word "touted" in the first sentence of the passage most nearly means
   a. praised
   b. denied
   c. exposed
   d. criticized

   Question type_____

ANSWERS AND EXPLANATIONS FOR PRACTICE PASSAGE 1

Don't just look at the right answers and move on. The explanations are the most important part, so read them carefully. Use these explanations to help you understand how to tackle each kind of question the next time you come across it.

1. b. Question type: 1, fact or detail. The passage says that community policing began "in the last decade." A decade is a period of ten years. In addition, the passage identifies 1983 as the first large-scale use of community policing in Houston. Don't be misled by trying to figure out when Carter was president. Also, if you happen to know that Lee Brown was New York City's police commissioner, don't let that information lead you away from the information contained in the passage alone. Brown was commissioner in Houston when he initiated community policing.

2. c. Question type: 3, inference. The "network of trust" referred to in this passage is between the community and the police, as you can see from the sentence where the phrase appears. The key phrase in the question is *in this passage.* You may think that police can rely only on each other, or one of the other answer choices may appear equally plausible to you. But your choice of answers must be limited to the one suggested *in this passage.* Another tip for questions like this: Beware of absolutes! Be suspicious of any answer containing words like *only, always,* or *never.*

3. d. Question type: 2, main idea. The title always expresses the main idea. In this passage, the main idea comes at the end. The sum of all the details in the passage suggests that community policing is not without its critics and that therefore its

future is uncertain. Another key phrase is *mixed results,* which means that some communities haven't had full success with community policing.

4. a. Question type: 4, vocabulary. The word *touted* is linked in this passage with the phrase *the best way to reform.* Most people would think that a good way to reform something is praiseworthy. In addition, the next few sentences in the passage describe the benefits of community policing. Criticism or a negative response to the subject doesn't come until later in the passage.

DETAIL AND MAIN IDEA QUESTIONS

Main idea questions and fact or detail questions are both asking you for information that's right there in the passage. All you have to do is find it.

DETAIL OR FACT QUESTIONS

In detail or fact questions, you have to identify a specific item of information from the test. This is usually the simplest kind of question. You just have to be able to separate important information from less important information. However, the choices may often be very similar, so you must be careful not to get confused.

Be sure you read the passage and questions carefully. In fact, it is usually a good idea to read the questions first, *before* you even read the passage, so you'll know what details to look out for.

MAIN IDEA QUESTIONS

The main idea of a passage, like that of a paragraph or a book, is what it is *mostly* about. The main idea is like an umbrella that covers all of the ideas and details in the passage, so it is usually something general, not specific. For example, in Practice Passage 1, question 3 asked you what title would be best for the passage, and the correct answer was "Community Policing: An Uncertain Future." This is the best answer because it's the only one that includes both the positive and negative sides of community policing, both of which are discussed in the passage.

Sometimes the main idea is stated clearly, often in the first or last sentence of the passage—the main idea is expressed in the *last* sentence of Practice Passage 1, for example. The sentence that expresses the main idea is often referred to as the **topic sentence**.

At other times, the main idea is not stated in a topic sentence but is *implied* in the overall passage, and you'll need to determine the main idea by inference. Because there may be much information in the passage, the trick is to understand what all that information adds up to—the gist of what the author wants you to know. Often some of the wrong answers on main idea questions are specific facts or details from the passage. A good way to test yourself is to ask, "Can this answer serve as a *net* to hold the whole passage together?" If not, chances are you've chosen a fact or detail, not a main idea.

PRACTICE PASSAGE 2: DETAIL AND MAIN IDEA QUESTIONS

Practice answering main idea and detail questions by working on the questions that follow this passage. Circle the answers to the questions, and then check your answers against the key that appears immediately after the questions.

There are three different kinds of burns: first degree, second degree, and third degree. It is important for firefighters to be able to recognize each of these types of burns so that they can be sure burn victims are given proper medical treatment. The least serious burn is the first-degree burn, which causes the skin to turn red but does not cause blistering. A mild sunburn is a good example of a first-degree burn, and, like a mild sunburn, first-degree burns generally do not require medical treatment other than a gentle cooling of the burned skin with ice or cold tap water. Second-degree burns, on the other hand, do cause blistering of the skin and should be treated immediately. These burns should be immersed in warm water and then wrapped in a sterile dressing or bandage. (Do not apply butter or grease to these burns; despite the old wives' tale, butter does *not* help burns heal and actually increases chances of infection.) If second-degree burns cover a large part of the body, then the victim should be taken to the hospital immediately for medical care. Third-degree burns are those that char the skin and turn it black, or burn so deeply that the skin shows white. These burns usually result from direct contact with flames and have a great chance of becoming infected. All third-degree burns should receive immediate hospital care. They should not be immersed in water, and charred clothing should not be removed from the victim. If possible, a sterile dressing or bandage should be applied to burns before the victim is transported to the hospital.

1. Which of the following would be the best title for this passage?
   a. Dealing with Third-Degree Burns
   b. How to Recognize and Treat Different Burns
   c. Burn Categories
   d. Preventing Infection in Burns

2. Second-degree burns should be treated with
   a. butter
   b. nothing
   c. cold water
   d. warm water

3. First-degree burns turn the skin
   a. red
   b. blue
   c. black
   d. white

4. Which of the following best expresses the main idea of the passage?
   a. There are three different types of burns.
   b. Firefighters should always have cold compresses on hand.
   c. Different burns require different types of treatment.
   d. Butter is not good for healing burns.

ANSWERS AND EXPLANATIONS FOR PRACTICE PASSAGE 2

1. b. A question that asks you to choose a title for a passage is a main idea question. This main idea is expressed in the second sentence, the topic sentence: "It is important for firefighters to be able to recognize each of these types of burns so that they can be sure burn victims are given proper treatment." Answer **b** expresses this idea and is the only title that encompasses all of the ideas expressed in the passage. Answer **a** is too limited; it deals only with one of the kinds of burns discussed in the passage. Likewise, answers **c** and **d** are also too limited. Answer **c** covers types of burns but not their treatment, and **d** deals only with preventing infection, which is only a secondary part of the discussion of treatment.

2. d. The answer to this fact question is clearly expressed in the sentence, "These burns should be immersed in warm water and then wrapped in a sterile dressing or bandage." The hard part is keeping track of whether "These burns" refers to the kind of burns in the question, which is second-

degree burns. It's easy to choose a wrong answer here because all of the answer choices are mentioned in the passage. You need to read carefully to be sure you match the right burn to the right treatment.

3. a. This is another fact or detail question. The passage says that a first-degree burn "causes the skin to turn red." Again, it's important to read carefully because all of the answer choices (except **b**, which can be eliminated immediately) are listed elsewhere in the passage.

4. c. Clearly this is a main idea question, and **c** is the only answer that encompasses the whole passage. Answers **b** and **d** are limited to *particular* burns or treatments, and answer **a** discusses only burns and not their treatment. In addition, the second sentence tells us that "It is important for firefighters to be able to *recognize each of these types of burns so that they can be sure burn victims are given proper medical treatment.*"

INFERENCE AND VOCABULARY QUESTIONS

Questions that ask you about the meaning of vocabulary words in the passage and those that ask what the passage *suggests* or *implies* (inference questions) are different from detail or main idea questions. In vocabulary and inference questions, you usually have to pull ideas from the passage, sometimes from more than one place in the passage.

INFERENCE QUESTIONS

Inference questions can be the most difficult to answer because they require you to draw meaning from the text when that meaning is implied rather than directly stated. Inferences are conclusions that we draw based on the clues the writer has given us. When you draw inferences, you have to be something of a detective, looking for such clues as word choice, tone, and specific details that suggest a certain conclusion, attitude, or point of view. You have to read between the lines in order to make a judgment about what an author was implying in the passage.

A good way to test whether you've drawn an acceptable inference is to ask, "What evidence do I have for this inference?" If you can't find any, you probably have the wrong answer. You need to be sure that your inference is logical and that it is based on something that is suggested or implied in the passage itself—not by what you or others might think. Like a good detective, you need to base your conclusions on evidence—facts, details, and other information—not on random hunches or guesses.

VOCABULARY QUESTIONS

Questions designed to test vocabulary are really trying to measure how well you can figure out the meaning of an unfamiliar word from its context. *Context* refers to the words and ideas surrounding a vocabulary word. If the context is clear enough, you should be able to substitute a nonsense word for the one being sought, and you would still make the right choice because you could determine meaning strictly from the sense of the sentence. For example, you should be able to determine the meaning of the italicized nonsense word below based on its context:

The speaker noted that it gave him great *terivinix* to announce the winner of the Outstanding Leadership Award.

In this sentence, *terivinix* most likely means

  a. pain
  b. sympathy
  c. pleasure
  d. anxiety

Clearly, the context of an award makes **c**, *pleasure*, the best choice. Awards don't usually bring pain, sympathy, or anxiety.

When confronted with an unfamiliar word, try substituting a nonsense word and see if the context gives you the clue. If you're familiar with prefixes, suffixes, and word roots, you can also use this knowledge to help you determine the meaning of an unfamiliar word.

You should be careful not to guess at the answer to vocabulary questions based on how you may have seen the word used before or what you *think* it means. Many words have more than one possible meaning, depending on the context in which they're used, and a word you've seen used one way may mean something else in a test passage. Also, if you don't look at the context carefully, you may make the mistake of confusing the vocabulary word with a similar word. For example, the vocabulary word may be *taut* (meaning *tight*), but if you read too quickly or don't check the context, you might think the word is *tout* (meaning *publicize* or *praise*) or *taunt* (meaning *tease*). Always make sure you read carefully and that what you think the word means fits into the context of the passage you're being tested on.

PRACTICE PASSAGE 3:
INFERENCE AND VOCABULARY QUESTIONS

The questions that follow this passage are strictly vocabulary and inference questions. Circle the answers to the questions, and then check your answers against the key that appears immediately after the questions.

Dealing with irritable patients is a great challenge for health-care workers on every level. It is critical that you do not lose your patience when confronted by such a patient. When handling irate patients, be sure to remember that they are not angry at you; they are simply projecting their anger at something else *onto* you. Remember that if you respond to these patients as irritably as they act with you, you will only increase their hostility, making it much more difficult to give them proper treatment. The best thing to do is to remain calm and ignore any imprecations patients may hurl your way. Such patients may be irrational and may not realize what they're saying. Often these patients will purposely try to anger you just to get some reaction out of you. If you react to this behavior with anger, they win by getting your attention, but you both lose because the patient is less likely to get proper care.

1. The word "irate" as it is used in the passage most nearly means
   a. irregular, odd
   b. happy, cheerful
   c. ill-tempered, angry
   d. sloppy, lazy

2. The passage suggests that health-care workers
   a. easily lose control of their emotions
   b. are better off not talking to their patients

   c. must be careful in dealing with irate patients because the patients may sue the hospital
   d. may provide inadequate treatment if they become angry at patients

3. An "imprecation" is most likely
   a. an object
   b. a curse
   c. a joke
   d. a medication

4. Which of the following best expresses the writer's views about irate patients?
   a. Some irate patients just want attention.
   b. Irate patients are always miserable.
   c. Irate patients should be made to wait for treatment.
   d. Managing irate patients is the key to a successful career.

ANSWERS AND EXPLANATIONS
FOR PRACTICE PASSAGE 3

1. **c.** This is a vocabulary question. *Irate* means *ill-tempered, angry*. It should be clear that **b**, *happy, cheerful*, is not the answer; dealing with happy patients is normally not "a great challenge." Patients that are **a**, *irregular, odd*, or **d**, *sloppy, lazy*, may be a challenge in their own way, but they aren't likely to rouse a health-care worker to anger. In addition, the passage explains that irate patients are not "*angry* at you," and *irate* is used as a synonym for *irritable*, which describes the patients under discussion in the very first sentence.

2. **d.** This is an inference question, as the phrase "the passage *suggests*" might have told you. The idea that angry health-care workers might give inadequate treatment is implied by the passage as a whole,

which seems to be an attempt to prevent angry reactions to irate patients. Furthermore, the last sentence in particular makes this inference possible: "If you react to this behavior with anger . . . you both lose because the patient is less likely to get proper care." Answer c is not correct, because while it may be true that some irate patients have sued the hospital in the past, there is no mention of suits anywhere in this passage. Likewise, answer b is incorrect; the passage does suggest ignoring patients' insults, but nowhere does it recommend not talking to patients—it simply recommends not talking angrily. And while it may be true that some health-care workers may lose control of their emotions, the passage does not provide any facts or details to support answer a, that they "*easily* lose control." Watch out for key works like *easily* that may distort the intent of the passage.

3. **b.** If you didn't know what an imprecation is, the context should reveal that it's something you can ignore, so neither **a**, an *object*, nor **d**, a *medication*, is a likely answer. Furthermore, **c** is not likely either, since an irate patient is not likely to be making jokes.

4. **a.** The writer seems to believe that some irate patients just want attention, as is suggested when the writer says, "Often these patients will purposely try to anger you just to get some reaction out of you. If you react to this behavior with anger, they win *by getting your attention*." It should be clear that **a** cannot be the answer, because it includes an absolute: "Irate patients are *always* miserable." Perhaps *some* of the patients are *often* miserable, but an absolute like *always* is almost always wrong. Besides, this passage refers to patients who may be irate in the hospital, but we have no indication of what these patients are like at other times, and *miserable* and *irate* are not exactly the same thing,

either. Answer **c** is also incorrect because the purpose of the passage is to ensure that patients receive "proper treatment" and that irate patients are not discriminated against because of their behavior. Thus, "irate patients should be made to wait for treatment" is not a logical answer. Finally, **d** cannot be correct because though it may be true, there is no discussion of career advancement in the passage.

REVIEW: PUTTING IT ALL TOGETHER

A good way to solidify what you've learned about reading comprehension questions is for *you* to write the questions. Here's a passage, followed by space for you to write your own questions. Write one question of each of the four types: fact or detail, main idea, inference, and vocabulary.

The "broken window" theory was originally developed to explain how minor acts of vandalism or disrespect can quickly escalate to crimes and attitudes that break down the entire social fabric of an area. It is a theory that can easily be applied to any situation in society. The theory contends that if a broken window in an abandoned building is not replaced quickly, soon all the windows will be broken. In other words, a small violation, if condoned, leads others to commit similar or greater violations. Thus, after all the windows have been broken, the building is likely to be looted and perhaps even burned down. According to this theory, violations increase exponentially. Thus, if disrespect to a superior is tolerated, others will be tempted to be disrespectful as well. A management crisis could erupt literally overnight. For example, if one firefighter begins to disregard proper housewatch procedure by neglecting to keep

If English Isn't Your First Language

When non-native speakers of English have trouble with reading comprehension tests, it's often because they lack the cultural, linguistic, and historical frame of reference that native speakers enjoy. People who have not lived in or been educated in the U.S. often don't have the background information that comes from reading American newspapers, magazines, and textbooks.

A second problem for non-native English speakers is the difficulty in recognizing vocabulary and idioms (expressions like "chewing the fat") that assist comprehension. In order to read with good understanding, it's important to have an immediate grasp of as many words as possible in the text. Test takers need to be able to recognize vocabulary and idioms immediately so that the ideas those words express are clear.

The Long View

Read newspapers, magazines, and other periodicals that deal with current events and matters of local, state, and national importance. Pay special attention to articles related to the career you want to pursue.

Be alert to new or unfamiliar vocabulary or terms that occur frequently in the popular press. Use a highlighter pen to mark new or unfamiliar words as you read. Keep a list of those words and their definitions. Review them for 15 minutes each day. Though at first you may find yourself looking up a lot of words, don't be frustrated—you'll look up fewer and fewer as your vocabulary expands.

During the Test

When you are taking the test, make a picture in your mind of the situation being described in the passage. Ask yourself, "What did the writer mostly want me to think about this subject?"

Locate and underline the topic sentence that carries the main idea of the passage. Remember that the topic sentence—if there is one—may not always be the first sentence. If there doesn't seem to be one, try to determine what idea summarizes the whole passage.

up the housewatch administrative journal, and this firefighter is not reprimanded, others will follow suit by committing similar violations of procedure, thinking, "If he can get away with it, why can't I?" So what starts out as a small thing, a violation that may seem not to warrant disciplinary action, may actually ruin the efficiency of the entire firehouse, putting the people the firehouse serves at risk.

1. Detail question:_____

   a.

   b.

   c.

   d.

2. Main idea question:_____
   a.
   b.
   c.
   d.

3. Inference question_____
   a.
   b.
   c.
   d.

4. Vocabulary question_____
   a.
   b.
   c.
   d.

POSSIBLE QUESTIONS

Here is one question of each type based on the passage above. Your questions may be very different, but these will give you an idea of the kinds of questions that could be asked.

1. Detail question: According to the passage, which of the following could happen "overnight"?
   a. The building will be burned down.
   b. The firehouse may become unmanageable.
   c. A management crisis might erupt.
   d. The windows will all be broken.

2. Main idea question: Which of the following best expresses the main idea of the passage?
   a. Even minor infractions warrant disciplinary action.

   b. Broken windows must be repaired immediately.
   c. People shouldn't be disrespectful to their superiors.
   d. Housewatch must be taken seriously.

3. Inference question: The passage suggests that
   a. the broken window theory is inadequate
   b. managers need to know how to handle a crisis
   c. firefighters are lazy
   d. people will get away with as much as they can

4. Vocabulary question: In this passage, *condoned* most nearly means
   a. punished
   b. overlooked
   c. condemned
   d. applauded

Answers
   1. c.
   2. a.
   3. d.
   4. b.

READING TABLES, GRAPHS, AND CHARTS

Depending on what position you're testing for, civil service exams may also include a section testing your ability to read tables, charts, and graphs. These sections are really quite similar to regular reading comprehension exams, but instead of pulling information from a passage of text, you'll need to answer questions about a graphic representation of data. The types of questions asked about tables, charts, and graphs are actually quite similar to those about reading passages, though there usually aren't any questions on vocabulary. The main difference in reading tables, charts, or graphs is that you're "reading" or interpreting data represented in tabular (table) or graphic (picture) form rather than textual (sentence and paragraph) form.

Tables

Tables present data in rows and columns. Here's a very simple table that shows the number of accidents reported in one county over a 24-hour period. Use it to answer the question that follows.

Time of Day	Number of Accidents
6:00 A.M.–9:00 A.M.	11
9:00 A.M.–12:00 P.M.	3
12:00 P.M.–3:00 P.M.	5
3:00 P.M.–6:00 P.M.	7
6:00 P.M.–9:00 P.M.	9
9:00 P.M.–12:00 A.M.	6
12:00 A.M.–3:00 A.M.	5
3:00 A.M.–6:00 A.M.	3

1. Based on the information provided in this table, at what time of day do the most accidents occur?
   a. noon
   b. morning rush hour
   c. evening rush hour
   d. midnight

The correct answer, of course, is **b**, morning rush hour. You can clearly see that the highest number of accidents (11) occurred between 6:00 A.M. and 9:00 A.M.

Graphs

Now, here's the same information presented as a graph. A graph uses two axes rather than columns and rows to create a visual picture of the data:

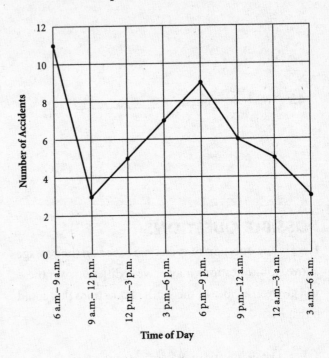

Here you can actually see the time of greatest number of accidents represented by a line that corresponds to the time of day and number. These numbers can also be represented by a box in a bar graph, as shown on the next page.

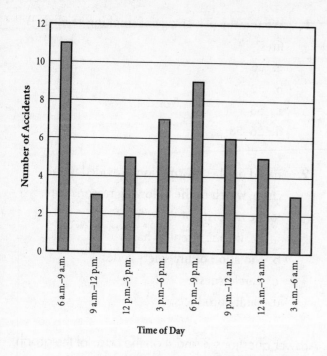

Time of Day

The key to "reading" graphs is to be sure that you know exactly what the numbers on each axis represent. Otherwise, you're likely to grossly misinterpret the information. Here, you see that the horizontal axis represents the time of day and the vertical axis represents the number of accidents that occurred. Thus, the tallest box shows the time of day with the most accidents.

Like regular reading comprehension questions, questions on tables, charts, and graphs may also ask you to make inferences and maybe even do basic math using the information and numbers the table, chart, or graph supplies. For example, you may be asked questions like the following on the information presented in the table, line graph, or bar graph above. The answers follow immediately after the questions.

2. What is the probable cause for the high accident rate between 6 A.M. and 9 A.M.?
   a. People haven't had their coffee yet.
   b. A lot of drivers are rushing to work.
   c. Sun glare.
   d. Construction.

3. What is the total number of accidents?
   a. 48
   b. 51
   c. 49
   d. 53

2. **b.** A question like this tests your common sense as well as your ability to read the graph. Though there may indeed be sun glare and though many drivers may not have had their coffee, these items are too variable to account for the high number of accidents. In addition, **d**, construction, is not logical because construction generally slows traffic down. Answer **b** is the best answer, because from 6:00 to 9:00 A.M. there is consistently a lot of rush hour traffic. In addition, many people do *rush*, and this increases the likelihood of accidents.

3. **c.** This question, of course, tests your basic ability to add. To answer this question correctly, you need to determine the value of each bar and then add those numbers together.

Charts

Finally, you may be presented information in the form of a chart like the pie chart on the next page. Here the accident figures have been converted to percentages. In this figure you don't see the exact number of accidents, but you see how accidents for each time period compare to the others.

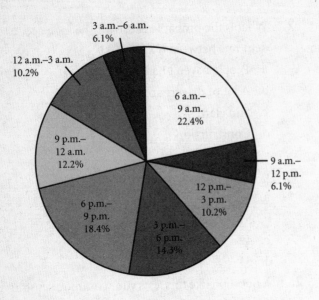

1. What is the percentage of smoking-related fires?
   a. 26
   b. 32
   c. 58
   d. 26–58

2. Based on the information provided in the chart, which of the following reasons applies to the majority of these fires?
   a. malicious intent to harm
   b. violation of fire safety codes
   c. carelessness
   d. faulty products

PRACTICE

Try the following questions to hone your skill at reading tables, graphs, and charts.

Answer questions 1 and 2 on the basis of the graph shown below.

Causes of household fires, in percentages

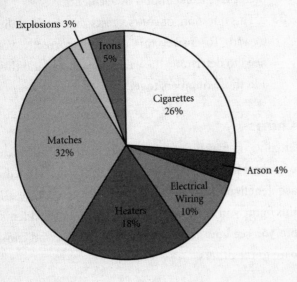

Answer questions 3 and 4 on the basis of the graph shown below.

Number of sick days per year of employment

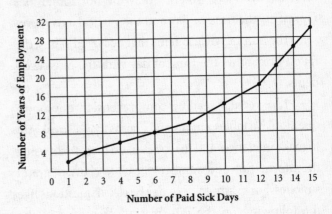

3. At what point does the rate of increase of sick days change?
   a. 4 years of employment
   b. 10 years of employment
   c. 8 years of employment
   d. 12 years of employment

4. During what years of employment are the number of sick days equal to double the number of years of employment?
  a. 1, 4, and 12
  b. 13, 14, and 15
  c. 1, 2, and 15
  d. 2, 4, and 10

ANSWERS AND EXPLANATIONS TO PRACTICE EXERCISE

1. d. Of the causes presented in the chart, both cigarettes (26 percent) and matches (32 percent) are related to smoking. But not all match fires are necessarily smoking related. Thus, the best answer allows for a range between 26 percent and 58 percent.

2. c. Fires from cigarettes, heaters, irons, and matches—81 percent in total—are generally the result of carelessness. Only 4 percent of fires are arsons, so **a** cannot be correct. Electrical, heater, and explosion fires *may* be the result of fire safety code violations, but even so, they total only 31 percent. Finally, there's no indication in this chart that there were faulty products involved.

3. b. In the first nine years, employees gain an additional two sick days every two years. At ten years of employment, however, the gain increases from two days every two years to four days, that is, from ten days in the eighth year to fourteen days in the tenth year.

4. c. In the first year, the number of sick days is two; in the second, four; and not until the fifteenth year does the number of sick days (thirty) again double the number of years of employment.

ADDITIONAL RESOURCES

Here are some other ways you can build the vocabulary and knowledge that will help you do well on reading comprehension questions.

- Practice asking the four sample question types about passages you read for information or pleasure.
- If you belong to a computer network such as America Online or Compuserve, search out articles related to the career you'd like to pursue. Exchange views with others on the Internet. All of these exchanges will help expand your knowledge of job-related material that may appear in a passage on the test.
- Use your library. Many public libraries have sections, sometimes called "Lifelong Learning Centers," that contain materials for adult learners. In these sections you can find books with exercises in reading and study skills. It's also a good idea to enlarge your base of information by reading related books and articles. Many libraries have computer systems that allow you to access information quickly and easily. Library personnel will show you how to use the computers and microfilm and microfiche machines.
- Begin now to build a broad knowledge of your potential profession. Get in the habit of reading articles in newspapers and magazines on job-related issues. Keep a clipping file of those articles. This will help keep you informed of trends in the profession and familiarize you with pertinent vocabulary.
- Consider reading or subscribing to professional journals or magazines.
- If you need more help building your reading skills and taking reading comprehension tests, consider *Reading Comprehension in 20 Minutes a Day* by Elizabeth Chesla, published by LearningExpress. Order information is in the back of this book.

C·H·A·P·T·E·R
VERBAL EXPRESSION
7

CHAPTER SUMMARY

This chapter will help you brush up your vocabulary and grammar skills so that you'll be able to do well on exam questions that test your ability to express yourself in writing.

Some questions on the sanitation worker exam test how well you can use words to express yourself. Basically, there are two different kinds of questions: **vocabulary** questions ask you to identify the meanings of words, while **clarity** questions ask you which is the best way to express the information given in the question.

Here's an example of a **vocabulary** question:

1. The mechanic inspected the hydraulic system and discovered that it was *defective*. This means that the system
   a. was in good working order
   b. needed to be recharged
   c. was not working properly
   d. was fully charged

The answer is **c**. Something that is *defective* contains a flaw that keeps it from working or looking as it should.

Clarity questions ask you to choose the sentence that states an idea most clearly and accurately.

2. A sanitation worker notices a leaking fire hydrant near 612 36th Street. This is between Woodland Avenue and Grand Avenue. Which of the following states the problem most clearly and accurately?
   a. The hydrant was leaking between Woodland and Grand Avenue. It's all wet and needs to be fixed.
   b. There's a leaking hydrant near 612 on 36th Street. That's between Grand and Woodland.
   c. At 612 between Grand and Woodland is a leaking hydrant.
   d. There's a leaking hydrant at Grand and Woodland at 36th Street. It's near 612.

The best answer is **b**. This answer choice states the problem and gives the exact location in the first sentence. It further identifies the location by mentioning the nearest cross streets.

This chapter explains in detail how to handle both vocabulary and clarity questions.

VOCABULARY

Many civil service exams test vocabulary. There are two basic kinds of questions.

- **Synonyms:** Identifying words that mean the same as the given words
- **Context:** Determining the meaning of a word or phrase by noting how it is used in a sentence or paragraph

SYNONYM QUESTIONS

A word is a *synonym* of another word if it has the same or nearly the same meaning as the other word. Test questions often ask you to find the synonym or antonym of a word. If you're lucky, the word will be surrounded by a sentence that helps you guess what the word means. If you're less lucky, you'll just get the word, and then you have to figure out what the word means without any help.

Questions that ask for synonyms can be tricky because they require you to recognize the meaning of several words that may be unfamiliar—not only the words in the questions but also the answer choices. Usually the best strategy is to *look* at the structure of the word and to *listen* for its sound. See if a part of a word looks familiar. Think of other words you know that have similar key elements. How could those words be related?

Synonym Practice

Try your hand at identifying the word parts and related words in these sample synonym questions. Circle the word that means the same or about the same as the italicized word. Answers and explanations appear right after the questions.

3. *incoherent* answer
   a. not understandable
   b. not likely
   c. undeniable
   d. challenging

4. *ambiguous* questions
   a. meaningless
   b. difficult
   c. simple
   d. vague

5. covered with *debris*
   a. good excuses
   b. transparent material
   c. scattered rubble
   d. protective material

6. *inadvertently* left
   a. mistakenly
   b. purposely
   c. cautiously
   d. carefully

7. *exorbitant* prices
   a. expensive
   b. unexpected
   c. reasonable
   d. outrageous

8. *compatible* workers
   a. gifted
   b. competitive
   c. harmonious
   d. experienced

9. *belligerent* attitude
   a. hostile
   b. reasonable
   c. instinctive
   d. friendly

Answers to Synonym Questions

The explanations are just as important as the answers, because they show you how to go about choosing a synonym if you don't know the word.

3. a. *Incoherent* means *not understandable*. To *cohere* means *to connect*. A coherent answer connects or makes sense. The prefix *in-* means *not*.

4. d. *Ambiguous* questions are *vague* or uncertain. The key part of this word is *ambi-*, which means *two* or *both*. An ambiguous question can be taken two ways.

5. c. *Debris* is scattered fragments and trash.

6. a. *Inadvertently* means *by mistake*. The key element in this word is the prefix *in-*, which usually means *not, the opposite of*.

7. d. The key element here is *ex-*, which means *out of* or *away from*. Exorbitant literally means "out of orbit." An *exorbitant* price would be an *outrageous* one.

8. c. *Compatible* means *harmonious*.

9. a. The key element in this word is the root *belli-*, which means *warlike*. The synonym choice, then, is *hostile*.

CONTEXT QUESTIONS

Context is the surrounding text in which a word is used. Most people use context to help them determine the meaning of an unknown word. A vocabulary question that gives you a sentence around the vocabulary word is usually easier to answer than one with little or no context. The surrounding text can help you as you look for synonyms for the specified words in the sentences.

The best way to take meaning from context is to look for key words in sentences or paragraphs that convey the meaning of the text. If nothing else, the context will give you a means to eliminate wrong answer choices that clearly don't fit. The process of elimination will often leave you with the correct answer.

Context Practice

Try these sample questions. Circle the word that best describes the meaning of the italicized word in the sentence.

10. The maintenance workers were *appalled* by the filthy, cluttered condition of the building.
   a. horrified
   b. amused
   c. surprised
   d. dismayed

11. Even though he seemed rich, the defendent claimed to be *destitute.*
 a. wealthy
 b. ambitious
 c. solvent
 d. poor

12. Though she was *distraught* over the disappearance of her child, the woman was calm enough to give the officer her description.
 a. punished
 b. distracted
 c. composed
 d. anguished

13. The evil criminal expressed no *remorse* for his actions.
 a. sympathy
 b. regret
 c. reward
 d. complacency

Some tests may ask you to fill in the blank by choosing a word that fits the context. In the following questions, circle the word that best completes the sentence.

14. Professor Washington was a very_____ man known for his reputation as a scholar.
 a. stubborn
 b. knowledgeable
 c. illiterate
 d. disciplined

15. His_____was demonstrated by his willingness to donate large amounts of money to worthy causes.
 a. honesty
 b. loyalty
 c. selfishness
 d. altruism

Answers to Context Questions

Check to see whether you were able to pick out the key words that help you define the target word, as well as whether you got the right answer.

10. **a.** The key words *filthy* and *cluttered* signify horror rather than the milder emotions described by the other choices.

11. **d.** The key word here is *rich,* but this is a clue by contrast. The introductory *Even though* signals that you should look for the opposite of the idea of having financial resources.

12. **d.** The key words here are *though* and *disappearance of her child,* signalling that you are looking for an opposite of *calm* in describing how the mother spoke to the officer. The only word strong enough to match the situation is *anguish.*

13. **b.** *Remorse* means *regret* for one's action. The part of the word here to beware of is the prefix *re-.* It doesn't signify anything in this word, though it often means again or back. Don't be confused by the two choices which also contain the prefix *re-.* The strategy here is to see which word sounds better in the sentence. The key words are *evil* and *no,* indicating that you're looking for something that shows no repentance.

14. **b.** The key words here are *professor* and *scholarly.*

15. **d.** The key words here are *large amounts of money to worthy causes.* They give you a definition of the word you're looking for. Even if you don't know the word *altruism,* the other choices seem inappropriate to describe someone so generous.

For Non-Native Speakers of English

Be very careful not to be confused by the *sound* of words that may mislead you. Be sure to look at the word carefully, and pay attention to the structure and appearance of the word as well as its sound. You may be used to hearing English words spoken with an accent. The sounds of those words may be misleading in choosing a correct answer.

WORD PARTS

The best way to improve your vocabulary is to learn word parts: roots, which are the main part of the word; prefixes, which go before the root word; or suffixes, which go after. Any of these elements can carry meaning or change the use of a word in a sentence. For instance, the suffix *-s* or *-es* can change the meaning of a noun from singular to plural: *boy, boys*. The prefix *un-* can change the meaning of a root word to its opposite: *necessary, unnecessary*.

On the next page are some of the word elements seen most often in vocabulary tests. Simply reading them and their examples five to ten minutes a day will give you the quick recognition you need to make a good association with the meaning of an unfamiliar word.

word element	meaning	example
ama	love	amateur
ambi	both	ambivalent, ambidextrous
aud	hear	audition
bell	war	belligerent, bellicose
bene	good	benefactor
cid/cis	cut	homicide, scissor
cogn/gno	know	knowledge, recognize
curr	run	current
flu/flux	flow	fluid, fluctuate
gress	to go	congress, congregation
in	not, in	ingenious
ject	throw	inject, reject
luc/lux	light	lucid, translucent
neo	new	neophyte
omni	all	omnivorous
pel/puls	push	impulse, propeller
pro	forward	project
pseudo	false	pseudonym
rog	ask	interrogate
sub	under	subjugate
spec/spic	look, see	spectator
super	over	superfluous
temp	time	contemporary, temporal
un	not, opposite	uncoordinated
viv	live	vivid

MORE VOCABULARY PRACTICE

Here is another set of practice exercises with samples of each kind of question covered in this chapter. Answers are at the end of the exercise.

Circle the word that means the same or nearly the same as the italicized word.

16. *congenial* company
- a. friendly
- b. dull
- c. tiresome
- d. angry

17. *conspicuous* mess
- a. secret
- b. notable
- c. visible
- d. boorish

18. *meticulous* record-keeping
- a. dishonest
- b. casual
- c. painstaking
- d. careless

19. *superficial* wounds
- a. life-threatening
- b. bloody
- c. severe
- d. surface

20. *impulsive* actions
- a. cautious
- b. sudden
- c. courageous
- d. cowardly

21. *tactful* comments
- a. polite
- b. rude
- c. angry
- d. confused

Using the context, choose the word that means the same or nearly the same as the italicized word.

22. Though flexible about homework, the teacher was *adamant* that papers be in on time.
- a. liberal
- b. casual
- c. strict
- d. pliable

23. The condition of the room after the party was *deplorable.*
- a. regrettable
- b. pristine
- c. festive
- d. tidy

Choose the word that best completes the following sentences.

24. Her position as a(n) _____ teacher took her all over the city.
- a. primary
- b. secondary
- c. itinerant
- d. permanent

25. Despite her promise to stay in touch, she remained _____ and difficult to locate.
- a. steadfast
- b. stubborn
- c. dishonest
- d. elusive

How to Answer Vocabulary Questions
- The key to answering vocabulary questions is to **notice and connect** what you do know to what you may not recognize.
- **Know your word parts.** You can recognize or make a good guess at the meanings of words when you see some suggested meaning in a root word, prefix, or suffix.
- **Use a process of elimination.** Think of how the word makes sense in the sentence.
- **Don't be confused by words that sound like other words,** but may have no relation to the word you need.

Answers to Practice Vocabulary Questions

16. a.
17. c.
18. c.
19. d.
20. b.
21. a.
22. c.
23. a.
24. c.
25. d.

CLARITY

Your communication skills may be tested in another way, by seeing how well you can express a given idea orally or in writing. You may be asked to read two or more versions of the same information and then choose the one that most clearly and accurately presents the given information, the **best** option. The **best** option should be:

- Accurate
- Clear
- Logical

Imagine this situation:

It is 2:30 on Tuesday, August 22. You are driving Vehicle #25, heading west on NW 91st Street. Your coworker Alex Thorp is riding on the platform at the back of the truck. Just as you round the corner to head north on Park Place, he loses his grip and falls from the truck. You stop immediately to see if he is hurt. He says he's fine, but about an hour later his wrist hurts badly enough that he asks you to take him to the hospital. You go to the Mercy Medical Center. The doctor who examines him says the wrist is mildly fractured.

The information above can be expressed accurately or inaccurately, clearly or unclearly, logically or illogically. The examples below will show you how this works.

ACCURATE

Check the facts for accuracy first. If the facts are wrong or confused in a particular answer choice, that choice is wrong, no matter how well written it is.

Inaccurate

Alex Thorp was in #25 on NE 91st when he fell off onto Park Place because he broke his wrist. I stopped, but he wasn't hurt. Later the doctor said he had a fractured wrist. It was 3:30 on Tuesday, August 22.

Accurate

Around 2:30 on Tuesday, August 22, Alex Thorp fell from the back platform of #25 while I was turning the corner from the west lane of NW 91st to go north on Park Place. About an hour later he asked to go to the hospital. The doctor said his wrist was fractured.

CLEAR

The best answer is written in plain English in such a way that most readers can understand it the first time through. If you read through an answer choice and then need to reread it to know what it means, look for a better option.

Garbled

On or about 2:30 on Tuesday, August 22, my coworker Alex Thorp and I were headed westbound on NW 91st Street. As I proceeded around the corner to head northbound on Park Place, he lost his grip and suffered an unknown injury. Later we went to Mercy Medical Center to seek a doctor's attention, who said it was fractured wrist, only mildly.

Clear

Around 2:30 on Tuesday, August 22, I was driving Vehicle #25, and Alex Thorp was riding on the back platform. He lost his grip and fell as I rounded a corner from NW 91st west onto Park Place north. He thought he was all right at first, but about an hour later he asked to go to the hospital. The doctor who saw him at Mercy Medical Center said he had a mildly fractured wrist.

LOGICAL

The best answer will present information in logical order, usually time order. If the information seems disorganized, look for a better option.

Illogical Order

The doctor said Alex's wrist was mildly fractured. It happened when he fell off the back of Vehicle #25. He went to the doctor later at Mercy Medical Center. It didn't hurt at first. He lost his grip. I turned from NW 91st west onto Park Place north. This was Tuesday, August 22, at around 2:30.

Logical Order

Around 2:30 on Tuesday, August 22, Alex Thorp lost his grip while riding on the back platform of Vehicle #25 as I was driving around the corner from NW 91st west onto Park Place north. He didn't realize he was hurt until about an hour later. I took him to Mercy Medical Center where a doctor examined him and said he had a mildly fractured wrist.

In addition to accuracy, clarity, and logic, below are some other characteristics of well-written sentences that you can look for.

MATCHING PRONOUNS

The **best** answer contains clearly identified pronouns (*he, she, him, her, them,* etc.) that match the number of nouns they represent. First, the pronouns should be clearly identified.

Unclear

Ann Dorr and the supervisor went to the central office, where she made her report.

Bob reminded his father that he had an appointment.

Clear

Ann Dorr and the supervisor went to the central office, where the supervisor made her report.

Bob reminded his father that Bob had an appointment.

An answer choice with clearly identified pronouns is a better choice than one with uncertain pronoun references. Sometimes the noun must be repeated to make the meaning clear.

In addition, the pronoun must match the noun it represents. If the noun is singular, the pronoun must be singular. Similarly, if the noun is plural, the pronoun must match.

Mismatch

I stopped the driver to tell them a headlight was burned out.

Match

I stopped the driver to tell him a headlight was burned out.

In the first example, *driver* is singular but the pronoun *them* is plural. In the second, the singular pronoun *him* matches the word it refers to.

CONSISTENT VERBS

The **best** option is one in which the verb tense is consistent. Look for answer choices that describe the action as though it has already happened, using past tense verbs (mostly *-ed* forms). The verb tense must remain consistent throughout the passage.

Inconsistent

I searched the cell and find nothing unusual.

Consistent

I searched the cell and found nothing unusual.

The verbs *opened* and *found* are both in the past tense in the second version. In the first, *find,* in the present tense, is inconsistent with *opened.*

It's easy to distinguish present tense from past tense by simply fitting the verb into a sentence.

VERB TENSE	
Present tense (Today, I ___...)	**Past Tense (Yesterday, I ___...)**
drive	drove
think	thought
rise	rose
catch	caught

The important thing to remember about verb tense is to keep it consistent. If a passage begins in the present tense, keep it in the present tense unless there is a specific reason to change—to indicate that some action occurred in the past, for instance. If a passage begins in the past tense, it should remain in the past tense.

Check yourself with these sample questions. Choose the option that uses verb tense correctly. The answers are right after the questions.

26.   a. When I cry, I always get what I want.
     b. When I cry, I always got what I want.
     c. When I cried, I always got what I want.
     d. When I cried, I always get what I wanted.

27.   a. It all started after I came home and am in my room studying for a big test.
     b. It all started after I came home and was in my room studying for a big test.
     c. It all starts after I come home and was in my room studying for a big test.
     d. It all starts after I came home and am in my room studying for a big test.

28.   a. The child became excited and dashes into the house and slams the door.
     b. The child becomes excited and dashed into the house and slammed the door.
     c. The child becomes excited and dashes into the house and slammed the door.
     d. The child became excited and dashed into the house and slammed the door.

Answers
26. a.
27. b.
28. d.

CLEAR MODIFIERS

The **best** option will use words clearly. Watch for unclear modifying words or phrases such as the ones in the following sentences. Misplaced and dangling modifiers can be hard to spot because your brain tries to make sense of things as it reads. In the case of misplaced or dangling modifiers, you may make a logical connection that is not present in the words.

Dangling Modifiers

Nailed to the tree, Cedric saw a "No Hunting" sign.
Waddling down the road, we saw a skunk.

Clear Modifiers

Cedric saw a "No Hunting" sign nailed to a tree.
We saw a skunk waddling down the road.

In the first version of the sentences, it sounds like *Cedric* was nailed to a tree and *we* were waddling down the road. The second version probably represents the writer's intentions: the *sign* was nailed to a tree and the *skunk* was waddling.

Misplaced Modifier

A dog followed the boy who was growling and barking.
George told us about safe sex in the kitchen.

Clear Modifiers

A dog who was growling and barking followed the boy.
In the kitchen, George told us about safe sex.

Do you think the boy was growling and barking? Did George discuss avoiding sharp knives and household poisons? The second version of each sentence represents the real situation.

EFFICIENT LANGUAGE

Finally, the **best** option will use words efficiently. Avoid answer choices that are redundant (repeat unnecessarily) or wordy. Extra words take up valuable time and increase the chances that facts will be misunderstood. In the following examples, the italicized words are redundant or unnecessary. Try reading the sentences without the italicized words.

Redundant

They refunded our money *back to us.*

We can proceed *ahead* with the plan we made *ahead of time.*

The car was red *in color.*

Wordy

The reason we left *was* because the job was done.

We didn't know what *it was* we were doing.

There are many citizens *who* obey the law.

In each case, the sentence is simpler and easier to read without the italicized words. When you find an answer choice that uses unnecessary words, look for a better option.

COMPLETE

The best option will be written in complete sentences. Sentences are the basic unit of written language. Most writing is done using complete sentences, so it's important to distinguish sentences from fragments. A sentence expresses a complete thought, while a fragment requires something more to express a complete thought.

Look at the word groups in the next column.

Fragment

The dog walking down the street.

Exploding from the bat for a home run.

Complete Sentence

The dog was walking down the street.

The ball exploded from the bat for a home run.

These examples show that a sentence must have a subject and a verb to complete its meaning. The first fragment has a subject but not a verb. *Walking* looks like a verb, but it is actually an adjective describing *dog*. The second fragment has neither a subject nor a verb. *Exploding* looks like a verb, but it actually describes something not identified in the word group.

Now look at the next set of word groups. Mark those that are complete sentences.

29. a. We saw the tornado approaching.
    b. When we saw the tornado approaching.

30. a. Before the house was built in 1972.
    b. The house was built in 1972.

31. a. Since we are leaving in the morning.
    b. We are leaving in the morning.

If you chose **29. a.**, **30.b.**, and **31.b.**, you were correct. You may have noticed that the groups of words are the same, but the fragments have an extra word at the beginning. These words are called subordinating conjunctions. If a group of words that would normally be a complete sentence is preceded by a subordinating conjunction, something more is needed to complete the thought.

■ When we saw the tornado approaching, we headed for cover.

- Before the house was built in 1972, the old house was demolished.
- Since we were leaving in the morning, we went to bed early.

Here is a list of words that can be used as subordinating conjunctions.

after	that
although	though
as	unless
because	until
before	when
if	whenever
once	where
since	wherever
than	while

SPECIFIC LANGUAGE

Language that is specific and detailed says more than language that is general and vague.

General

My sister and I enjoyed each other's company as we were growing up. We had a lot of fun, and I will always remember her. We did interesting things and played fun games.

Specific

As children, my sister and I built rafts out of old barrels and tires, then tried to float them on the pond behind our house. I'll never forget playing war or hide-and-seek in the grove beside the pond.

The idea behind both of these versions is similar, but the specific example is more interesting and memorable. Choose the option that uses specific language.

CORRECT WORDS

The best answer uses words correctly. The following word pairs are often misused in written language. By reading the explanations and looking at the examples, you can learn to spot the correct way of using these easily confused word pairs.

Its/it's

Its is a possessive pronoun that means "belonging to it." *It's* is a contraction for *it is* or *it has*. The only time you will ever use *it's* is when you can also substitute the words *it is* or *it has*.

Who/that

Who refers to people. *That* refers to things.

- There is the man *who* helped me find a new pet.
- The woman *who* invented the copper-bottomed kettle died in 1995.
- This is the house *that* Harold bought.
- The magazine *that* I needed was no longer in print.

There/their/they're

Their is a possessive pronoun that shows ownership. *There* is an adverb that tells where an action or item is located. *They're* is a contraction for the words *they are*. Here is an easy way to remember these words.

- *Their* means "belonging to them." Of the three words, *their* can be most easily transformed into the word *them*. Extend the *r* on the right side and connect the *i* and the *r* to turn *their* into *them*. This clue will help you remember that *their* means "belonging to them."
- If you examine the word *there*, you can see from the way it's written that it contains the word *here*. Whenever you use *there*, you should be able to

substitute *here*. The sentence should still make sense.

- Imagine that the apostrophe in *they're* is actually a very small letter *a*. Use *they're* in a sentence only when you can substitute *they are*.

Your/you're

Your is a possessive pronoun that means "belonging to you." *You're* is a contraction for the words *you are*. The only time you will ever use *you're* is when you can also substitute the words *you are*.

To/too/two

To is a preposition or an infinitive.

- As a preposition: to the mall, to the bottom, to my church, to our garage, to his school, to his hideout, to our disadvantage, to an open room, to a ballad, to the gymnasium
- As an infinitive (*to* followed by a verb, sometimes separated by adverbs): to walk, to leap, to see badly, to find, to advance, to read, to build, to sorely want, to badly misinterpret, to carefully peruse

Too means "also." Whenever you use the word *too*, substitute the word *also*. The sentence should still make sense.

Two is a number, as in one, two. If you give it any thought at all, you'll never misuse this form.

The key is to think consciously about these words when you see them in written language. Circle the correct form of these easily confused words in the following sentences. Answers are at the end of the exercise.

32. (Its, It's) (to, too, two) late (to, too, two) remedy the problem now.

33. This is the man (who, that) helped me find the book I needed.

34. (There, Their, They're) going (to, too, two) begin construction as soon as the plans are finished.

35. We left (there, their, they're) house after the storm subsided.

36. I think (your, you're) going (to, too, two) win at least (to, too, two) more times.

37. The corporation moved (its, it's) home office.

Answers

32. It's, too, to
33. who
34. They're, to
35. their
36. you're, to, two
37. its

Following are four sample multiple-choice questions. By applying the principles explained in this section, choose the best version of each of the four sets of sentences. The answers and a short explanation for each question follow the exercise.

38. a. Vanover caught the ball. This was after it had been thrown by the shortstop. Vanover was the first baseman who caught the double-play ball. The shortstop was Hennings. He caught a line drive.
   b. After the shortstop Hennings caught the line drive, he threw it to the first baseman Vanover for the double play.
   c. After the line drive was caught by Hennings, the shortstop, it was thrown to Vanover at first base for a double play.

d. Vanover the first baseman caught the flip from shortstop Hennings.

39. a. This writer attended the movie *Casino* starring Robert DeNiro.
b. The movie *Casino* starring Robert DeNiro was attended by me.
c. The movie *Casino* starring Robert DeNiro was attended by this writer.
d. I attended the movie *Casino* starring Robert DeNiro.

40. a. They gave cereal boxes with prizes inside to the children.
b. They gave cereal boxes to children with prizes inside.
c. Children were given boxes of cereal by them with prizes inside.
d. Inside the boxes of cereal were prizes. The children got them.

41. a. After playing an exciting drum solo, the crowd rose to its feet and then claps and yells until the band plays another cut from their new album.
b. After playing an exciting drum solo, the crowd rose to its feet and then clapped and yelled until the band played another cut from their new album.
c. After the drummer's exciting solo, the crowd rose to its feet and then claps and yells until the band plays another cut from their new album.
d. After the drummer's exciting solo, the crowd rose to its feet and then clapped and yelled until the band played another cut from their new album.

The BEST Option
- Is accurate
- Is written in plain English
- Presents information in a logical order
- Has clearly identified pronouns that match the number of the nouns they represent
- Has a consistent verb tense
- Uses modifiers clearly
- Uses words efficiently
- Is written using complete sentences
- Is specific
- Uses words correctly

Answers

38. b. Answer **a** is unnecessarily wordy and the order is not logical. Answer **c** is also wordy and unclear. Answer **d** omits a piece of important information.

39. d. Both answers **a** and **c** use the stuffy-sounding *this writer.* Answer **d** is best because it avoids the wordy phrase "was attended by."

40. a. In both answers **b** and **c** the modifying phrase *with prizes inside* is misplaced.

41. d. Both answers **a** and **b** contain a dangling modifier, stating that the crowd played an exciting drum solo. Both answers **b** and **c** mix past and present verb tense. Only answer **d** has clearly written modifiers and a consistent verb tense.

ADDITIONAL RESOURCES

One of the best resources for any adult student is the public library. Many libraries have sections for adult learners or for those preparing to enter or change careers. Those sections contain skill books and review books on a number of subjects, including vocabulary. Here are some books you might consult:

- *504 Absolutely Essential Words* by Murray Bromberg et al. (Barron's)
- *All About Words: An Adult Approach to Vocabulary Building* by Maxwell Nurnberg and Morris Rosenblum (Mentor Books)
- *Checklists for Vocabulary Study* by Richard Yorkey (Longman)
- *Vocabulary and Spelling in 20 Minutes a Day* by Judith Meyers (LearningExpress, order information at the back of this book)
- *Word Watcher's Handbook* by Phyllis Martin (St. Martin's)
- *Word Smart Revised* by Adam Robinson (The Princeton Review)

- *The Handbook of Good English* by Edward D. Johnson (Washington Square Press)
- *Smart English* by Anne Francis (Signet)
- *Writing Smart* by Marcia Lerner (Princeton Review)

For more help with verbal expression, here are some books you can consult.

For Non-Native Speakers of English
- *English Made Simple* by Arthur Waldhorn and Arthur Ziegler (Made Simple Books)
- *Errors in English and How to Correct Them* by Harry Shaw (HarperCollins)
- *Living in English* by Betsy J. Blusser (National Textbook Company)

For Everyone
- *Better English* by Norman Lewis (Dell)
- *Writing Skills in 20 Minutes a Day* by Judith Olson (LearningExpress, order information at the back of this book)
- *1001 Pitfalls in English Grammar* (Barron's)

C·H·A·P·T·E·R 8

MAP READING AND SPATIAL RELATIONS

CHAPTER SUMMARY

This chapter shows you how to do well on civil service examinations that ask you to answer questions about maps or other spatial representations.

If you don't have a "sense of direction," the time is ripe to develop one. Sanitation workers need to be on friendly terms with maps in order to be successful. That north-south-east-west thing can be confusing, but with a little practice you'll be picking out the most efficient, quickest way to get around, both in real life and when you see map questions on the civil service exam. Practice is the only way to get good at map reading.

Once you get to where you need to be, even more decisions must be made. Is the collection truck you are driving going to make it down that crowded street without peeling off a few side mirrors on parked cars? Is it better to carry that old sofa between the two parked cars, or walk around the cars to the space that looks a little bigger? When you are faced with this kind of situation you are dealing with spatial relations—and it's something you probably do every day without ever giving it a thought. Civil service exams have given it some thought, though, and they came up with a way to test both your map-reading and spatial skills.

MAP READING

Map reading questions come with a simple map with the north-south-east-west directions clearly marked and a key explaining symbols. You'll find instructions on which questions should be answered based on the map.

A sentence or two is usually devoted to telling you that you can't make up your own traffic laws in order to get from Point A to Point B. You can't go up one-way streets the wrong way or choose paths that will have you driving through office buildings. After that, you'll find one or more questions about the map you're looking at. The questions may ask you which is the shortest route from Point A to Point B, or they may tell you to make a series of right and left turns and then ask you in which direction you're heading.

FINDING THE SHORTEST ROUTE

Questions that ask you to find the shortest legal route are based on a map like the one on the next page. A scenario follows the instructions, followed by a question asking for the shortest route and the answer choices.

The best approach to solving these puzzles is to first study the map for a minute to get your bearings. Read the question, then turn to the map and figure out what looks like the best route to you. (Do not look at the answers before figuring out the route you would take.) Start with the first answer choice and study each route turn-by-turn. If none of the options looks like the route you came up with after first reading the question, then you may need to reconsider your route. If this is the case, then you'll also need to start over and consider all of the options with a fresh eye. Try this strategy on the sample question that follows.

Sample Shortest-Route Question

Here's a question that asks you to find the shortest route on the map on the next page.

Answer Questions 1 through 3 based solely on the following map. You are required to follow traffic laws and the flow of traffic. A single arrow depicts one-way streets and two arrows pointing in opposite directions represent two-way streets.

1. Sanitation Worker Ali, the collection truck driver, has a route sheet that tells her to start her collections route on Second Street. The route sheet states that she must start at the corner of River Road and Second Street, and she is now on Ash Road just east of Fourth Street. What is the safest, most direct legal route for Ali to take?
   a. Turn north on Church Street, then west on Main Street, and then north on Second Street to River Road.
   b. Turn south on Church Street, then west on McArthur Boulevard, north on Parker Road, and then east on River Road to Second Street.
   c. Turn north on Church Street and west on River Road to Second Street.
   d. Turn north on Church Street, then west on Washington Road, north on Third Street, and west on River Road to Second Street.

Strategy for Shortest-Route Questions

Here's how to apply the strategy outlined above for this question.

Look at the map carefully to get used to how the streets run. Keep in mind that you are not allowed to break traffic laws to get where you need to be. Watch those arrows that show you which streets are one way

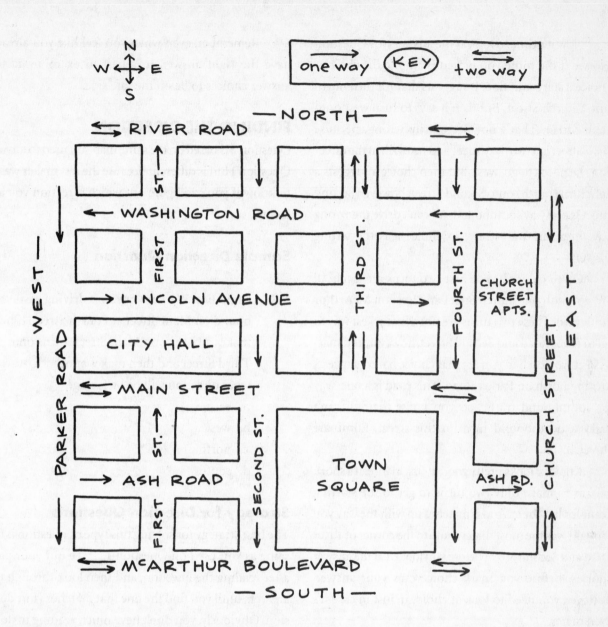

and which are two way. The question tells you that Sanitation Worker Ali is on Ash Road east of Fourth Street. You find Ash Road on the map and should note that this road is a one-way for traffic to flow east; therefore, Ali is headed east on Ash Road between Fourth and Church Streets. Church Street is a two-way street, so you know that Ali can turn left (north) or right (south) on this street.

Now look for the destination. Ali has to get to the corner of River Road and Second Street. River Road is at the top of the map (north) and is a two-way street. So when you start planning the route, you'll probably want Ali to turn north on Church Street, not south. Thus, the most direct route for Ali to take to River Road and Second Street is to go north on Church Street until she gets to River Road and then make a left (west) turn on River Road. Second Street, which is a one-way street, is only three blocks away. From River Road, Ali will be able to turn left (south) onto Second Street. Ali is ready to start her route as far as you're concerned.

Now it's time to look at the answers for Question 1 to see if the route you picked is among the choices. Choice **a** starts out fine. It suggests that Ali turn north onto Church Street. But then it says to turn west onto Main Street. That's not necessarily wrong, because Main Street is a two-way street and takes Ali in the direction she needs to go, west. But then choice **a** suggests a right turn (north) onto Second Street; however, Second Street is one way southbound. Ali can't drive the wrong way on a one-way street, so choice **a** is the wrong answer.

On to choice **b**. The first two turns are legal: Ali can go south on Church Street and west on McArthur Boulevard. These two turns are not the quickest way to get to River Road and Second Street, however, and matters get worse when you see that choice **b** next suggests turning north on Parker Road. This road is a one-way for southbound traffic, so you know that Ali can't make a northbound turn on this street. Eliminate choice **b**.

Choice **c** looks pretty good at first glance. It's short; Ali has to make only two turns to get to the starting point for her route. And it matches up with the way you thought was the most direct route to the corner of River Road and Second Street before you looked at the answer choices. Before you mark choice **c** as your answer, however, you need to look at choice **d**, just in case it's even better.

You soon find that choice **d** is a much less direct route than choice **c**. It does not suggest any illegal turns as the first two choices did, but it does require Ali to make too many turns. It's far easier to make two turns in a large collection vehicle down crowded city streets than it is to make four turns—and that means it's safer, too, to keep the number of turns down to as few as possible.

Remember, even when you feel like you already have the right answer, it is best to examine *all* the answer choices to be on the safe side.

FINDING THE DIRECTION

Question 2 is based on the same map you used to answer Question 1 but is different because the test maker wants to know if you can figure out which direction you are facing.

Sample Direction Question

2. Sanitation Worker Watson is driving eastbound on Main Street at Fourth Street. If he makes a U-turn on Main Street, turns onto Third Street and then makes another U-turn, what direction will he be facing?
   a. east
   b. west
   c. north
   d. south

Strategy for Direction Questions

The best strategy for solving this type of question is the same as you used on Question 1. Trace out your path after reading the question, and then look through the answers until you find the one that matches your decision. Obviously, you don't have much reading to do to pick out the right answer. You'll mainly be looking to see which letter is in front of the answer you want.

In the case of Question 2, the answer you want is **d**. When you traced out your path on the map, you should have seen that if Watson is heading east on Main Street and he makes a U-turn, he will be heading west. If he turns onto Third Street, the only way he can turn will have him heading north on Third Street. If he makes a second U-turn, he will now be facing south.

MORE MAP-READING PRACTICE

The key to answering map-reading questions is to *take your time*. If you hurry through a question you may misread the question or the answer choices, which will naturally cause you to choose the wrong answer.

Let's try a third question using the same sample map.

3. On an icy day, Sanitations Workers Epps and Burton are dispatched to spread sand starting at Ash Road and Church Street. They are driving north on First Street and have just passed Washington Road. What is the quickest route they can take?
   a. North on First Street, west on River Road, south on Parker Road, east on McArthur Boulevard, and then north on Church Street to Ash Road.
   b. North on First Street, east on River Road, south on Third Street, east on Main Street, and then north on Church Street to Ash Road.
   c. North on First Street, east on River Road, and then south on Church Street to Ash Road.
   d. North on First Street, west on River Road, south on Parker Road, east on Lincoln Avenue, south on Second Street, east on

McArthur Boulevard, and then north on Church Street to Ash Road.

After reading the question you are ready to trace your route. Keep in mind that you want to get to Ash Road and Church Street in the quickest, easiest manner without going the wrong way on any one-way streets. First Street is a one-way street going toward a two-way street, River Road. You have the option of heading east or west on River Road. East makes more sense because it is in the direction of Church Street. The most direct route appears to be east on River Road to Church Street, and then south on Church Street to Ash Road.

Now it's time to check your answer against the options. Option **a** has you turning west on First Street, and you've already determined that west is not the most efficient direction to turn. Option **b** suggests that you turn east on River Road, then south on Third Street, then east on Main Street, and then north on Church Street. You should turn south on Church Street to get to Ash Road, not north. You already have too many turns for this to be an efficient route in any event. Time to look at option **c**. Option **c** directs you east on River Road, then south on Church Street—and there you are at Ash Road. This route matches the route we had in mind. Option **d** has too many turns (like option **b**), in addition to involving a west turn onto River Road, which we already decided was inefficient.

Tips for Map-Reading Questions

- Read carefully and follow all directions.
- Feel free to move the map around during the test to face the direction you find comfortable.
- Trace your path lightly on the map with your pencil. Make sure you erase all marks as you complete each question so that you do not confuse yourself for the next question.

Now that you're becoming an expert in map reading, be sure to make up your own questions to test your growing skills.

SPATIAL RELATIONS

Now you have a pretty good idea how to get where you are going, at least as far as a written test is concerned. Another, similar kind of question is concerned with what you do when you get there. Spatial relations questions test your ability to judge distances between objects, shapes, and sizes of objects. The answer choices may be expressed in words, in which case you have to visualize the objects described in your head, or you may be asked to choose your answers from simple drawings.

Most of these questions may seem simple, and basically they are. That's why it's especially important for you to read them *carefully*. You could get tripped up by such words and phrases as *best*, *most likely*, or *least likely*. Pay close attention to what the question asks.

Distances

You may see a test question that asks you to judge whether or not an object you are carrying can fit through a narrow space. This kind of question may come with a diagram of a street, like the one in the next column.

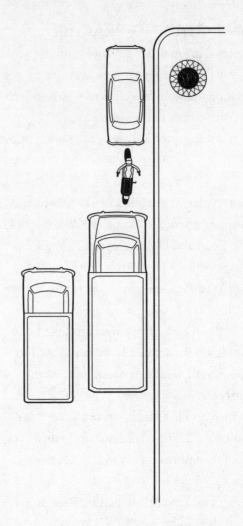

4. You and your partner are collecting trash from wire basket containers on street corners. A car, a motorcycle, and a delivery truck are illegally parked in your way. The container is too full and heavy to carry over your head. Which of the following is the best way for you to carry the container back to the truck?
   a. between the motorcycle and the car
   b. behind the delivery truck
   c. between the motorcycle and the delivery truck
   d. in front of the car

Looking at the diagram, you can see that there is not room to walk between any of the vehicles—at least, not while carrying the containers—so **a** and **c** are not good choices. Choice **d** would make you walk into the traffic at the corner and is the longest path to the back of the collection vehicle. That leaves choice **b** as the best choice.

Shapes

Another type of question may ask you to pick which object you think will be the easiest for a sanitation worker to carry to a collection truck. You may have to choose an answer from four drawings, which is a little easier, or from a description of the objects, which is a little harder. If the answer choices are words rather than pictures, as in the example below, you'll have to visualize the objects in order to answer the question.

5. Which object would a sanitation worker most easily be able to roll to the collection truck without assistance?
    a. the top of a round wooden table without its legs
    b. a box of broken picture frames
    c. an end table with one corner broken off
    d. an upholstered easy chair

Obviously, the closer something is to being round, the easier it will be to roll. So you try to visualize the four objects described to see which one is closest to being round. Choice **a** is the best choice because a sanitation worker would be able to roll the table top the way a child rolls a hoop. The other objects aren't round. A box of broken picture frames is not likely to roll. Neither is a table that has corners or a chair.

Sizes

Other types of spatial relations questions may ask you to differentiate between sizes of items you might be required to pick up on your collection route. This type, too, might use either words or pictures. Here's one that uses pictures:

6. You are driving a collection truck that is almost completely full. You think you may have space for one more object, but only if it is very small. Of the objects below, which is most likely to fit in the space you have left under these circumstances?

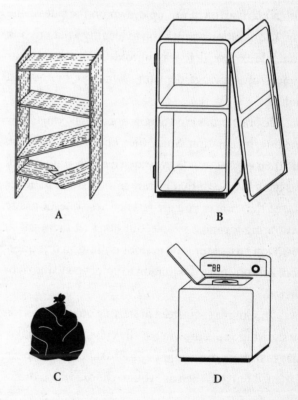

A

B

C

D

    a. object A
    b. object B
    c. object C
    d. object D

The question asks you to think small—to pick out the smallest of the four objects you see listed. Choice **c** should stand out as the smallest of all the objects. Once again, the "catch" lies in how well you read the question. If you rush through a question because it looks easy, you risk overlooking a key phrase. The key phrase above is *most likely.*

Dimensions

There's one more type of question, one you may have experienced at one time or another. This kind of question tests your ability to visualize a two-dimensional picture as a three-dimensional object. You might, for instance, be shown a drawing of a cube (or little box) with a black arrow point up drawn on the side of the box. The question will ask you to identify what this box would look like if it was unfolded. You'd see four choices of drawings depicting what the box would look like.

To answer this kind of question, you'll need to rely on your imagination. Study the cube or box for a bit, and then in your mind's eye watch it slowly unfold until it is lying flat. See if that picture in your mind matches one of the choices you are given. These questions are frustrating for most people, but don't let them get to you. Don't dwell for long periods of time on one question. Rely on your visualization to point you to the right answer.

In some cases, instead of starting out the question by showing you a drawing of the cube, the test maker may first show you a cube or other shape that has been flattened out and then ask you to choose which draw-

ing you think is correct *after* the cube has been folded up. It's the reverse of the above example. So, instead of visualizing yourself unfolding the cube, you will simply visualize yourself folding the cube up. The technique remains the same.

Instead of identifying the cube folded or unfolded, you may be shown a drawing of an object facing one direction and then be asked to pick out this same object facing a different direction. The object may not necessarily be in the shape of a cube. The object may be upside down, facing left, facing right, or maybe even shown lying on its side. Your strategy is the same as what you'd do for the cube drawings: visualization. Turn the figure in your mind's eye in every direction until you can pick out one of the four choices as being your original object facing a different direction. Don't worry. It's much easier than it sounds and you'll find examples to practice with in the practice exam.

THE SAME, YET DIFFERENT

Map reading and spatial relations may not seem to have much in common when you first think about it, but they both rely on your ability to visualize situations and objects in your mind. Folding a cube in your mind is a lot like visualizing turns on a map in your mind. The skills you use will be very much the same.

This is where you'll need your self-confidence and patience. Psyching yourself up for this kind of exam is important. *You* know you can do it. Now it's time to show *them* you can do it. Practice these skills and go to it!

GOOD JUDGMENT AND COMMON SENSE

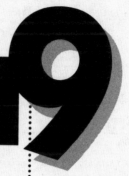

CHAPTER SUMMARY

This chapter shows you how to deal with exam questions that test your judgment and common sense. Reading carefully and learning to think like a sanitation worker are the keys to doing well on these questions.

ompetition for decently paying jobs is pretty stiff and isn't likely to let up any time soon. One of the most sought-after jobs for men and women without much formal education is that of sanitation worker. You might not need a college degree to get one of the positions, but you *will* need a big helping of common sense and good judgment, as well as decent driving skills. These qualities are what it takes to keep smiles on the faces of taxpayers and city supervisors.

Multiple-choice civil service exams are the quickest, most cost-effective way for city officials to find applicants with common sense and good judgment. These exams feature judgment questions that reveal whether you can make a sound decision—pick the right multiple-choice answer—based on the information given to you. To come to the right conclusion, you will need your common sense, good judgment, and good reading skills. (A little good luck never hurts either, so feel free to stick that four-leaf clover in your pocket.)

Judgment questions usually fall into three categories: judgment based on routine or emergency situations, judgment based on public relations, and application of rules and procedures. This chapter will look at each category, take apart an example of each type of judgment question, and then identify the best approach to answering the question. There are also tips on what is most likely to trip up the unwary test-taker.

JUDGMENT IN ROUTINE OR EMERGENCY SITUATIONS

Situational judgment questions ask you to climb inside the mind of a sanitation worker and make decisions from this viewpoint. It isn't necessary for you to know sanitation department policies or technical information about operating a collection vehicle. The test itself will give you the information you need to answer the question.

Some exams load you right into the hot seat with language such as "You are collecting in a residential neighborhood when. . ." while other exams use a more subtle approach: "Sanitation Worker Jones is operating a street sweeper when she sees a school bus stopped ahead." Although the approach is different, both test makers are asking you to look at their questions from the same viewpoint—a sanitation worker's view.

The structure of the questions is pretty simple. You'll be given a situation, and then you'll be asked to choose how you would handle the situation if you were the sanitation worker. The nice part is that you don't have to come up with your own plan. You get to choose the best answer from four multiple-choice options listed below the question. Eye-bulging panic, of course, will make all of the options appear to be the right one, but keep in mind that there is only *one* best answer.

Here's an example:

1. You are driving a collection vehicle in rush-hour traffic when you notice that the truck is pulling hard to the right. You stop the truck and see that the right front tire is almost flat. What should you do?
   a. ignore the tire and finish the route on the bare rim if necessary
   b. turn on your hazard lights and change the tire
   c. drive more slowly for the rest of your run
   d. use the truck radio to call for assistance

Now would be a good time to pull out the common sense and good judgment skills. Put yourself in the driver's seat and look at this situation. The question tells you two things: it's rush hour, and you have a potentially dangerous problem with your vehicle. Keep this in mind as you read the four options.

Option a is not a good choice. Driving on the tire rim will damage the truck and make steering hazardous. Option b is not a good choice. You wouldn't be able to change the tire without special equipment, and even if you could, doing it in rush-hour traffic would be impractical and dangerous. Option c is also not a good choice. If you ignored the tire and continued your run, you would be jeopardizing your own safety as well as the safety of other drivers who have to share the street with you. That leaves option d as the wisest choice. Stopping your route and calling for assistance may put you behind schedule a bit, but this choice makes the most sense—the most *common* sense

Along with using common sense and good judgment, you are using another tool to answer this question—the process of elimination. As you read each option, you make a decision about whether you want to eliminate this possibility or keep it. Sometimes even if you don't know for sure where the right answer is, you can find it by pitching out all the wrong ones.

The temptation with situational judgment questions is to project your thoughts and feelings into the scenario. You may catch yourself chewing on your pencil thinking, "Well, I'd drive to the nearest service station. That's what I would do." That may be how this situation would play out in real life, but that's not one of your options, so this kind of thinking merely complicates the question.

Another temptation is to read more into the situation than is there. You may think, "Maybe the tire isn't all that flat...." Use the information you *see on the page*, not the information that *could* be there, to make your decision.

THROUGH THEIR EYES

It's easy to say "think like a sanitation worker" if you know how sanitation workers think. The ideal way to learn is to watch sanitation workers at work and see how they handle their jobs. Do what you can to look at the world through their eyes.

After you see for yourself what sanitation workers do, then arm yourself with the next few paragraphs.

Safety First

If your momma always told you "safety first" when you went out to play as a child, then you are well-trained for *this* job. The safety and well-being of everyone around you is Priority Number One—yes, even including the rude drivers who glare when they have to wait to go around your street sweeper.

The safety issue pops up in judgment questions fairly often. As you read the questions during the test, keep the "Safety First" motto in the forefront of your mind. If you think this way, the right answer may suddenly stand out as if it were in bold print. Ask yourself, "How does this situation affect my safety or the safety of others?" If you asked yourself this question when you answered the sample question above, then you probably eliminated all the wrong choices without a second thought, keeping only the one that kept you and your

vehicle safe. Any answer that places anyone in danger is not going to be the one you want.

Medical Emergencies

Along with safety issues, some of the questions on the test may deal with medical emergency situations. Consider the following example:

2. Your coworker, who is walking toward the collection vehicle, trips and hits his head on the edge of the truck as he falls. He is unconscious on the ground when you check on him. What action should you take?
   a. don't move him, and call on the truck radio for medical assistance
   b. pick him up, prop him by the curb, and wait for him to wake up
   c. pour cold water on him to wake him up
   d. elevate his feet and wait for him to wake up

You may be thinking to yourself that this is not a fair question because you wouldn't be able to pick out the right answer unless you knew all about first aid. Well, that's the very reason this question is an easy question. The only option that mentions calling for help is option **a**, and your common sense should tell you that you will need to call for help under these conditions. If you also happen to know a little first aid, you may have realized that you shouldn't move your coworker because you could make any possible neck or back injuries worse.

That's why option **b** is not a good choice: You should never move someone when you do not know the extent of the injuries. Option **c** is not a good choice because, while pouring water on an unconscious victim may look good on the movie screen, it's not something you'd want to do in the real world: the victim could choke. Option **d** is not a good choice because elevating your coworker's feet involves moving him. It's best to leave the coworker where he is until help arrives, unless you can tell, of course, that the way he is positioned creates a life-threatening situation (for instance, he can't breathe). Getting help should be your first priority, and that's why a is the best choice.

Most people have been exposed to basic first aid principles at school or work or even through television. Just in case they've slipped your mind, here are a few short, easy-to-learn rules that may make answering emergency medical situation questions much easier.

- Before you do anything else, call for help.
- Don't move an injured person unless fire or some other life-threatening situation endangers the victim.
- If you have been trained, begin cardiopulmonary resuscitation (CPR) if the injured person is not breathing.
- If an injured person is bleeding, apply direct pressure to the wound with your hand or a clean cloth. Keep the pressure on until help arrives.
- Don't give an injured person anything to drink, not even if the person asks for water.
- To keep shock from setting in, keep the injured person covered with a coat or blanket until help arrives.
- If live electrical wires are involved, do not touch the injured person or the vehicle the victim is in. Tell the victim not to move until help arrives.

Physical Contact

In a medical emergency, a certain amount of physical contact with the victim may be necessary. Touching people is not always a good idea, however. Whenever you see an option in a multiple-choice question that suggests you come into physical contact with a civilian, you'll want to look at that option closely, and most times

you should reject it. Touching a civilian who does not consent to that contact—for instance, during a disagreement—can open you up to a lawsuit and/or minor criminal charges. Common sense strongly recommends that you keep your hands to yourself—especially in our lawsuit-happy society. So, if one of the options in a question suggests that you touch a civilian (other than in an emergency situation), keep the liability issue in mind when picking your answer.

JUDGMENT IN PUBLIC RELATIONS

Some questions may deal not so much with routine or emergency situations as with your relationships with customers. You'll be asked to choose the answers that show you have the ability to use good judgment in a situation that will have an impact on how customers view both you and sanitation department in general. For example, suppose you see the following question:

3. You are running behind schedule on your route in a residential neighborhood. As you finish picking up in front of a group of private houses, you see an elderly woman coming toward you dragging a full trash can. Suddenly, the woman turns over the can. She is struggling to turn it right side up. What should you do?
   a tell her to hurry
   b. walk to meet her and take the can from her
   c. get in the truck and drive away, since you can take her garbage on the next pickup day
   d. shout to her that she has to have the garbage on the curb before you arrive and then leave without taking her garbage

Option a is rude and does nothing to solve the problem. Option c is also rude. You can indeed take her garbage on the next run, but leaving while this woman is struggling to bring you her garbage is hardly good public relations. Option **d** provokes the same reaction as option **c**. Thus, your best choice is option **b**. Helping an elderly person with her garbage is humane and professional behavior.

Simply put, this kind of question will test how you relate to the public. Can you make choices that will demonstrate that you can get along with others and treat people with respect? This is what the test maker *and* your potential employer want to know.

Tips for Answering Situational Judgment Questions

- Read carefully, but don't read anything into the situation that isn't there.
- Think like a sanitation worker: Safety first.
- Use your common sense.
- Be polite.

APPLICATION OF RULES AND PROCEDURES

Another kind of test question asks you to read rules, laws, policies, or procedures and then apply those guidelines to a hypothetical situation. You might have to decide which step in a set of procedures is the next step to be taken in the situation, or you might have to decide whether a hypothetical sanitation worker followed the procedures properly in the situation given. In either case, you're being tested on your ability to follow directions, including your reading comprehension skills.

The question is usually preceded by a brief passage telling you about the procedure; for example:

When a sanitation worker discovers valuable property that may have been lost or discarded accidentally, the worker should follow these procedures:

1. Fill out a Found Property Slip stating what the object is, where it was found, and who found it.

2. Place the property in a safe area near the driver's seat until the end of the shift.

3. Turn in the property to the shift supervisor at the end of the shift.

4. Turn one copy of the Found Property Slip with the property and keep the other for personal files.

4. Sanitation Worker Enrico is halfway through his shift when he finds a woman's purse on top of a pile of trash in a wire basket on a busy street corner. He sees that the purse contains credit cards, money, identification, and other valuables. Enrico fills out a Found Property slip and puts the purse in the cab of the vehicle. What should he do at the end of the day?
    a. fill out a leave request slip
    b. use the identification in the purse to call the owner
    c. turn in the purse to his supervisor along with one copy of the Found Property slip
    d. return to the street corner where he found the purse and wait to see if the woman shows up

What the test maker wants you to do is study how Enrico handled the found property case and see what he should do to follow his department's rules on handling found property.

One way to approach picking the right choice is to see if you can assign a step to the information in one of the lettered choices. For example, option **a** states that

Enrico should fill out a leave request slip. If you go back to the text above the sample question, you will not see filling out a leave request listed as a step anywhere in the procedure. So this is one way to tell that a is not going to be the right answer. You can apply the same technique to options b and d and get the same result. Option c, on the other hand, is the right answer because you can see that handing in both the property and the slip is listed as step 4.

Another hint that should point you in the right direction is the phrase "What should he do at the end of the day?" Step 4 states exactly what Enrico should do.

Tips for Answering Application Questions

- Read what's there, not what might have been there.
- Read through all the options before you choose an answer.
- Find the spot in the rule or procedure that supports your answer.

IMPROVING YOUR JUDGMENT SKILLS

You have more options than you may realize when it comes to honing your judgment skills—not only for the exam, but also for your job as a sanitation worker. There are some surprisingly simple exercises you can do in your everyday life that will get you ready.

WHAT IF . . .

Exam preparation is not *all* work. There's a game you can play in your mind that will help you prepare for the test. It's called "What If." You've played before, but you may not have been aware of it. "What if I won the lottery tomorrow? If I did, I'd empty my desk drawers on top of my supervisor's desk and run screaming out of the building." Sound familiar?

Some professional baseball players watch slow-motion videos of a batter with perfect form in the hope that by memorizing and studying his moves, they will be able to improve their own performance. And research shows that this works: In times of stress, people are more likely to carry out a task if they've practiced it—mentally or physically.

You can use the same idea in preparing to think like a sanitation worker. Find out when collection service takes place on your street and take time to watch how the sanitation worker handles his or her job. Say to yourself, "What would I do if I was driving that collection truck and my partner needed help picking up that broken refrigerator?" Then decide how you'd handle it. The situation you dream up, and the solution, may be one you see on the test, or it might be what happens to you when you are driving your own route some day.

If you've thought about a situation and arrived at a conclusion about what you would do under the circumstances, you've given your brain a plan of action for when the situation actually arises. Practice. You'll be helping yourself for the exam *and* for your job.

SELF-CONFIDENCE CHECKS

Practice your self-confidence. Odd advice? Not really. Self-confidence is what makes most people able to make decisions with a minimum of confusion and self-doubt. You need self-confidence so that you will make the right decisions as a test taker. If you aren't confident about your judgment skills and your ability to decide what to do in a situation, then you are likely to torture yourself with every judgment question.

Believe it or not, it is possible to practice self-confidence. Many people practice the opposite of self-confidence by thinking and saying things like "I don't know if I can do that" or "What if I can't do that?"

Start listening to yourself to see if you talk like that. And then turn it around. Tell yourself and others, "The civil service test is coming up and I intend to ace it." And "I know I will make a good sanitation worker. I know that when I read the test questions I can rely on my own good judgment to help me. My common sense will point me in the right direction."

This isn't bragging. It's how you set yourself up for success. You'll start thinking of what you need to do to ace the test. You're practicing self-confidence right now by reading this book. You are getting the tools you need to do the job. Your self-confidence has no option but to shoot straight up—and your score along with it.

READ, READ, READ

Reading is as vital on judgment questions as it is on questions that call themselves reading questions. This isn't the kind of reading you do when you are skimming a novel or skipping through articles in a newspaper. It's the kind where you not only have to pay attention to what the writer is telling you, but you must make decisions based on the information you've received. There's a whole chapter in this book on reading. Check it out.

MATH

10

CHAPTER SUMMARY

This chapter gives you some important tips for dealing with math questions on a civil service exam and reviews some of the most commonly tested concepts. If you've forgotten most of your high school math or have math anxiety, this chapter is for you.

Not all civil service exams test your math knowledge, but many do. Knowledge of basic arithmetic, as well as the more complex kinds of reasoning necessary for algebra and geometry problems, are important qualifications for almost any profession. You have to be able to add up dollar figures, evaluate budgets, compute percentages, and other such tasks, both in your job and in your personal life. Even if your exam doesn't include math, you'll find that the material in this chapter will be useful on the job.

The math portion of the test covers the subjects you probably studied in grade school and high school. While every test is different, most emphasize arithmetic skills and word problems.

MATH STRATEGIES

- **Don't work in your head!** Use your test book or scratch paper to take notes, draw pictures, and calculate. Although you might think that you can solve math questions more quickly in your head, that's a good way to make mistakes. Write out each step.
- **Read a math question in *chunks*** rather than straight through from beginning to end. As you read each *chunk,* stop to think about what it means and make notes or draw a picture to represent that *chunk.*
- **When you get to the actual question, circle it.** This will keep you more focused as you solve the problem.
- **Glance at the answer choices for clues.** If they're fractions, you probably should do your work in fractions; if they're decimals, you should probably work in decimals; etc.
- **Make a plan of attack** to help you solve the problem.
- **If a question stumps you, try one of the *backdoor* approaches** explained in the next section. These are particularly useful for solving word problems.
- **When you get your answer, reread the circled question to make sure you've answered it.** This helps avoid the careless mistake of answering the wrong question.
- **Check your work after you get an answer.** Test-takers get a false sense of security when they get an answer that matches one of the multiple-choice answers. Here are some good ways to check your work *if you have time:*
  - Ask yourself if your answer is reasonable, if it makes sense.
  - Plug your answer back into the problem to make sure the problem holds together.
  - Do the question a second time, but use a different method.
- **Approximate when appropriate.** For example:
  - $5.98 + $8.97 is a little less than $15. (Add: $6 + $9)
  - $.9876 \times 5.0342$ is close to 5. (Multiply: 1×5)
- **Skip hard questions and come back to them later.** Mark them in your test book so you can find them quickly.

BACKDOOR APPROACHES FOR ANSWERING QUESTIONS THAT PUZZLE YOU

Remember those word problems you dreaded in high school? Many of them are actually easier to solve by backdoor approaches. The two techniques that follow are terrific ways to solve multiple-choice word problems that you don't know how to solve with a straightforward approach. The first technique, *nice numbers*, is useful when there are unknowns (like x) in the text of the word problem, making the problem too abstract for you. The second technique, *working backwards*, presents a quick way to substitute numeric answer choices back into the problem to see which one works.

Nice Numbers

1. When a question contains unknowns, like x, plug nice numbers in for the unknowns. A nice number is easy to calculate with and makes sense in the problem.

2. Read the question with the nice numbers in place. Then solve it.

3. If the answer choices are all numbers, the choice that matches your answer is the right one.

4. If the answer choices contain unknowns, substitute the same nice numbers into **all** the answer choices. The choice that matches your answer is the right one. If more than one answer matches, do the problem again with different nice numbers. You'll only have to check the answer choices that have already matched.

Example: Judi went shopping with p dollars in her pocket. If the price of shirts was s shirts for d dollars, what is the maximum number of shirts Judi could buy with the money in her pocket?

a. psd **b.** $\frac{ps}{d}$ **c.** $\frac{pd}{s}$ **d.** $\frac{ds}{p}$

To solve this problem, let's try these nice numbers: $p = \$100$, $s = 2$; $d = \$25$. Now reread it with the numbers in place:

Judi went shopping with *$100* in her pocket. If the price of shirts was *2* shirts for *$25*, what is the maximum number of shirts Judi could buy with the money in her pocket?

Since 2 shirts cost $25, that means that 4 shirts cost $50, and 8 shirts cost $100. So our answer is *8*. Let's substitute the nice numbers into all 4 answers:

a. $100 \times 2 \times 25 = 5000$ **b.** $\frac{100 \times 2}{25} = 8$ **c.** $\frac{100 \times 25}{2} = 1250$ **d.** $\frac{25 \times 2}{100} = \frac{1}{2}$

The answer is **b** because it is the only one that matches our answer of **8**.

Working Backwards

You can frequently solve a word problem by plugging the answer choices back into the text of the problem to see which one fits all the facts stated in the problem. The process is faster than you think because you'll probably only have to substitute one or two answers to find the right one.

This approach works only when:

- All of the answer choices are numbers.
- You're asked to find a simple number, not a sum, product, difference, or ratio.

Here's what to do:

1. Look at all the answer choices and begin with the one in the middle of the range. For example, if the answers are 14, 8, 2, 20, and 25, begin by plugging 14 into the problem.

2. If your choice doesn't work, eliminate it. Determine if you need a bigger or smaller answer.

3. Plug in one of the remaining choices.

4. If none of the answers work, you may have made a careless error. Begin again or look for your mistake.

Example: Juan ate $\frac{1}{3}$ of the jellybeans. Maria then ate $\frac{3}{4}$ of the remaining jellybeans, which left 10 jellybeans. How many jellybeans were there to begin with?

a. 60 **b.** 80 **c.** 90 **d.** 120 **e.** 140

Starting with the middle answer, let's assume there were **90** jellybeans to begin with:

Since Juan ate $\frac{1}{3}$ of them, that means he ate 30 ($\frac{1}{3} \times 90 = 30$), leaving 60 of them ($90 - 30 = 60$). Maria then ate $\frac{3}{4}$ of the 60 jellybeans, or 45 of them ($\frac{3}{4} \times 60 = 45$). That leaves 15 jellybeans ($60 - 45 = 15$).

The problem states that there were **10** jellybeans left, and we wound up with **15** of them. That indicates that we started with too big a number. Thus, 90, 120, and 140 are all wrong! With only two choices left, let's use common sense to decide which one to try. The next lower answer is only a little smaller than 90 and may not be small enough. So, let's try **60**:

Since Juan ate $\frac{1}{3}$ of them, that means he ate 20 ($\frac{1}{3} \times 60 = 20$), leaving 40 of them ($60 - 20 = 40$). Maria then ate $\frac{3}{4}$ of the 40 jellybeans, or 30 of them ($\frac{3}{4} \times 40 = 30$). That leaves 10 jellybeans ($40 - 30 = 10$).

Because this result of **10** jellybeans left agrees with the problem, the right answer is **a**.

WORD PROBLEMS

Many of the math problems on tests are word problems. A word problem can include any kind of math, including simple arithmetic, fractions, decimals, percentages, even algebra and geometry.

The hardest part of any word problem is translating English into math. When you read a problem, you can frequently translate it *word for word* from English statements into mathematical statements. At other times, however, a key word in the word problem hints at the mathematical operation to be performed. Here are the translation rules:

EQUALS   key words: **is, are, has**

English	Math
Bob **is** 18 years old.	B = 18
There **are** 7 hats.	H = 7
Judi **has** 5 books.	J = 5

ADDITION   key words: **sum; more, greater, or older than; total; altogether**

English	Math
The **sum** of two numbers is 10.	X + Y = 10
Karen has $5 **more than** Sam.	K = 5 + S
The base is 3″ **greater than** the height.	B = 3 + H
Judi is 2 years **older than** Tony.	J = 2 + T
The **total** of three numbers is 25.	A + B + C = 25
How much do Joan and Tom have **altogether**?	J + T = ?

SUBTRACTION   key words: **difference, less or younger than, remain, left over**

English	Math
The **difference** between two numbers is 17.	X + Y = 17
Mike has 5 **less** cats **than** twice the number Jan has.	M = 2J − 5
Jay is 2 years **younger than** Brett.	J = B − 2
After Carol ate 3 apples, R apples **remained**.	R = A − 3

MULTIPLICATION   key words: of, product, times

English	Math
20% **of** Matthew's baseball caps	$.20 \times M$
Half **of** the boys	$\frac{1}{2} \times B$
The **product** of two numbers is 12	$A \times B = 12$

DIVISION   key word: per

English	Math
15 drops **per** teaspoon	$\frac{15 \text{ drops}}{\text{teaspoon}}$
22 miles **per** gallon	$\frac{22 \text{ miles}}{\text{gallon}}$

DISTANCE FORMULA: DISTANCE = RATE × TIME

The key words are movement words like: plane, train, boat, car, walk, run, climb, swim

- How far did the **plane** travel in 4 hours if it averaged 300 miles per hour?

  $D = 300 \times 4$

  $D = 1200$ miles

- Ben **walked** 20 miles in 4 hours. What was his average speed?

  $20 = r \times 4$

  5 miles per hour = r

SOLVING A WORD PROBLEM USING THE TRANSLATION TABLE

Remember the problem at the beginning of this chapter about the jellybeans?

Juan ate $\frac{1}{3}$ of the jellybeans. Maria then ate $\frac{3}{4}$ of the remaining jellybeans, which left 10 jellybeans. How many jellybeans were there to begin with?

| **a.** 60 | **b.** 80 | **c.** 90 | **d.** 120 | **e.** 140 |

We solved it by *working backwards*. Now let's solve it using our translation rules.

Assume Juan started with J jellybeans. Eating $\frac{1}{3}$ of them means eating $\frac{1}{3} \times J$ jellybeans. Maria ate a fraction of the **remaining** jellybeans, which means we must **subtract** to find out how many are left: $J - \frac{1}{3} \times J = \frac{2}{3} \times J$. Maria then ate $\frac{3}{4}$, leaving $\frac{1}{4}$ of the $\frac{2}{3} \times J$ jellybeans, or $\frac{1}{4} \times \frac{2}{3} \times J$ *jellybeans. Multiplying out* $\frac{1}{4} \times \frac{2}{3} \times J$ gives $\frac{1}{6}J$ as the number of jellybeans Maria ate. Altogether, Juan and Maria ate $\frac{1}{3}J + \frac{1}{2}J$ jellybeans , or $\frac{5}{6}J$ jellybeans. Add the number of jellybeans they both ate to the 10 leftover jellybeans to get the number of jelly beans they started with.

$$\frac{5}{6}J + 10 = J$$
$$10 = J - \frac{5}{6}J$$
$$10 = \frac{1}{6}J$$
$$60 = J$$

Solving this equation for *J* gives *J* = **60**. Thus, the right answer is **a** (the same answer we got when we *worked backwards*). As you can see, both methods—working backwards and translating from English to math—work. You should use whichever method is more comfortable for you.

PRACTICE WORD PROBLEMS

You will find word problems using fractions, decimals, and percentages in those sections of this chapter. For now, practice using the translation table on problems that just require you to work with basic arithmetic. Answers are at the end of the chapter.

_____ **1.** Joan went shopping with $100 and returned home with only $18.42. How much money did she spend?

    a. $81.58   **b.** $72.68   **c.** $72.58   **d.** $71.68   **e.** $71.58

_____ **2.** Mark invited ten friends to a party. Each friend brought 3 guests. How many people came to the party, excluding Mark?

    a. 3   **b.** 10   **c.** 30   **d.** 40   **e.** 41

_____ **3.** The office secretary can type 80 words per minute on his word processor. How many minutes will it take him to type a report containing 760 words?

    a. 8   **b.** $8\frac{1}{2}$ **c.** 9   **d.** $9\frac{1}{2}$ **e.** 10

_____ **4.** Mr. Wallace is writing a budget request to upgrade his personal computer system. He wants to purchase 4 mb of RAM, which will cost $100, two new software programs at $350 each, a tape backup system for $249, and an additional tape for $25. What is the total amount Mr. Wallace should write on his budget request?

    a. $724   **b.** $974   **c.** $1049   **d.** $1064   **e.** $1074

FRACTION REVIEW

Problems involving fractions may be straightforward calculation questions, or they may be word problems. Typically, they ask you to add, subtract, multiply, divide, or compare fractions.

WORKING WITH FRACTIONS

A fraction is a part of something.

Example: Let's say that a pizza was cut into 8 equal slices and you ate 3 of them. The fraction $\frac{3}{8}$ tells you what part of the pizza you ate. The pizza below shows this: 3 of the 8 pieces (the ones you ate) are shaded.

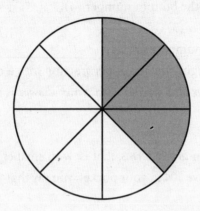

Three Kinds of Fractions

Proper fraction: The top number is less than the bottom number:

$\frac{1}{2}$; $\frac{2}{3}$; $\frac{4}{9}$; $\frac{8}{13}$

The value of a proper fraction is less than 1.

Improper fraction: The top number is greater than or equal to the bottom number:

$\frac{3}{2}$; $\frac{5}{3}$; $\frac{14}{9}$; $\frac{12}{12}$

The value of an improper fraction is 1 or more.

Mixed number: A fraction written to the right of a whole number:

$3\frac{1}{2}$; $4\frac{2}{3}$; $12\frac{3}{4}$; $24\frac{3}{4}$

The value of a mixed number is more than 1: it is the sum of the whole number plus the fraction.

Changing Improper Fractions into Mixed or Whole Numbers

It's easier to add and subtract fractions that are mixed numbers rather than improper fractions. To change an improper fraction, say $\frac{13}{2}$, into a mixed number, follow these steps:

1. Divide the bottom number (2) into the top number (13) to get the whole number portion (6) of the mixed number:

$$\begin{array}{r} 6 \\ 2\overline{)13} \\ \underline{12} \\ 1 \end{array}$$

2. Write the remainder of the division (1) over the old bottom number (2): $6\frac{1}{2}$

3. Check: Change the mixed number back into an improper fraction (see steps below).

Changing Mixed Numbers into Improper Fractions

It's easier multiply and divide fractions when you're working with improper fractions rather than mixed numbers. To change a mixed number, say $2\frac{3}{4}$, into an improper fraction, follow these steps:

1. Multiply the whole number (2) by the bottom number (4). $\qquad$ $2 \times 4 = 8$

2. Add the result (8) to the top number (3). $\qquad$ $8 + 3 = 11$

3. Put the total (11) over the bottom number (4). $\qquad$ $\frac{11}{4}$

4. Check: Reverse the process by changing the improper fraction into a mixed number. If you get back the number you started with, your answer is right.

Reducing Fractions

Reducing a fraction means writing it in *lowest terms*, that is, with smaller numbers. For instance, 50¢ is $\frac{50}{100}$ of a dollar, or $\frac{1}{2}$ of a dollar. In fact, if you have 50¢ in your pocket, you say that you have half a dollar. Reducing a fraction does not change its value.

Follow these steps to reduce a fraction:

1. Find a whole number that divides *evenly* into both numbers that make up the fraction.

2. Divide that number into the top of the fraction, and replace the top of the fraction with the quotient (the answer you got when you divided).

3. Do the same thing to the bottom number.

4. Repeat the first 3 steps until you can't find a number that divides evenly into both numbers of the fraction.

For example, let's reduce $\frac{8}{24}$. We could do it in 2 steps: $\frac{8 \div 4}{24 \div 4} = \frac{2}{6}$; then $\frac{2 \div 2}{6 \div 2} = \frac{1}{3}$. Or we could do it in a single step: $\frac{8 \div 8}{24 \div 8} = \frac{1}{3}$.

Shortcut: When the top and bottom numbers both end in zeroes, cross out the same number of zeroes in both numbers to begin the reducing process. For example, $\frac{300}{4000}$ reduces to $\frac{3}{40}$ when you cross out 2 zeroes in both numbers.

Whenever you do arithmetic with fractions, reduce your answer. On a multiple-choice test, don't panic if your answer isn't listed. Try to reduce it and then compare it to the choices.

Reduce these fractions to lowest terms:

_____ **5.** $\frac{3}{12}$

_____ **6.** $\frac{14}{35}$

_____ **7.** $\frac{27}{72}$

Raising Fractions to Higher Terms

Before you can add and subtract fractions, you have to know how to raise a fraction to higher terms. This is actually the opposite of reducing a fraction.

Follow these steps to raise $\frac{2}{3}$ to 24ths:

1. Divide the old bottom number (3) into the new one (24): $3\overline{)24} = 8$
2. Multiply the answer (8) by the old top number (2): $2 \times 8 = 16$
3. Put the answer (16) over the new bottom number (24): $\frac{16}{24}$
4. Check: Reduce the new fraction to see if you get back the original one: $\frac{16 \div 8}{24 \div 8} = \frac{2}{3}$

Raise these fractions to higher terms:

_____ **8.** $\frac{5}{12} = \frac{}{24}$

_____ **9.** $\frac{2}{9} = \frac{}{27}$

_____ **10.** $\frac{2}{5} = \frac{}{500}$

ADDING FRACTIONS

If the fractions have the same bottom numbers, just add the top numbers together and write the total over the bottom number.

Examples: $\frac{2}{9} + \frac{4}{9} = \frac{2+4}{9} = \frac{6}{9}$ Reduce the sum: $\frac{2}{3}$

               $\frac{5}{8} + \frac{7}{8} = \frac{12}{8}$ Change the sum to a mixed number: $1\frac{4}{8}$; then reduce: $1\frac{1}{2}$

There are a few extra steps to add mixed numbers with the same bottom numbers, say $2\frac{3}{5} + 1\frac{4}{5}$:

1. Add the fractions: $\frac{3}{5} + \frac{4}{5} = \frac{7}{5}$
2. Change the improper fraction into a mixed number: $\frac{7}{5} = 1\frac{2}{5}$
3. Add the whole numbers: $2 + 1 = 3$
4. Add the results of steps 2 and 3: $1\frac{2}{5} + 3 = 4\frac{2}{5}$

Finding the Least Common Denominator

If the fractions you want to add don't have the same bottom number, you'll have to raise some or all of the fractions to higher terms so that they all have the same bottom number, called the **common denominator**. All of the original bottom numbers divide evenly into the common denominator. If it is the smallest number that they all divide evenly into, it is called the **least common denominator (LCD)**.

Here are a few tips for finding the LCD, the smallest number that all the bottom numbers evenly divide into:

- See if all the bottom numbers divide evenly into the biggest bottom number.
- Check out the multiplication table of the largest bottom number until you find a number that all the other bottom numbers evenly divide into.

- When all else fails, multiply all the bottom numbers together.

   Example: $\frac{2}{3} + \frac{4}{5}$

1. Find the LCD. Multiply the bottom numbers: $3 \times 5 = 15$

2. Raise each fraction to 15ths:
$$\frac{2}{3} = \frac{10}{15}$$
$$+\ \frac{4}{5} = \frac{12}{15}$$

3. Add as usual:
$$\frac{22}{15}$$

Try these addition problems:

_____**11.** $\frac{3}{4} + \frac{1}{6}$

_____**12.** $\frac{7}{8} + \frac{2}{3} + \frac{3}{4}$

_____**13.** $4\frac{1}{3} + 2\frac{3}{4} + \frac{1}{6}$

SUBTRACTING FRACTIONS

If the fractions have the same bottom numbers, just subtract the top numbers and write the difference over the bottom number.

   Example: $\frac{4}{9} - \frac{3}{9} = \frac{4-3}{9} = \frac{1}{9}$

   If the fractions you want to subtract don't have the same bottom number, you'll have to raise some or all of the fractions to higher terms so that they all have the same bottom number, or LCD. If you forgot how to find the LCD, just read the section on adding fractions with different bottom numbers.

   Example: $\frac{5}{6} - \frac{3}{4}$

1. Raise each fraction to 12ths because 12 is the LCD, the smallest number
   that 6 and 4 both divide into evenly:
$$\frac{5}{6} = \frac{10}{12}$$
$$-\ \frac{3}{4} = \frac{9}{12}$$

2. Subtract as usual:
$$\frac{1}{12}$$

   Subtracting mixed numbers with the same bottom number is similar to adding mixed numbers.

   Example: $4\frac{3}{5} - 1\frac{2}{5}$

1. Subtract the fractions: $\frac{3}{5} - \frac{2}{5} = \frac{1}{5}$

2. Subtract the whole numbers: $4 - 1 = 3$

3. Add the results of steps 1 and 2: $\frac{1}{5} + 3 = 3\frac{1}{5}$

   Sometimes there is an extra "borrowing" step when you subtract mixed numbers with the same bottom numbers, say $7\frac{3}{5} - 2\frac{4}{5}$:

1. You can't subtract the fractions the way they are because $\frac{4}{5}$ is bigger than $\frac{3}{5}$.

So you borrow 1 from the 7, making it 6, and change that 1 to $\frac{5}{5}$ because

5 is the bottom number: $\qquad\qquad\qquad\qquad\qquad\qquad 7\frac{3}{5} = 6\frac{5}{5} + \frac{3}{5}$

2. Add the numbers from step 1: $\qquad\qquad\qquad\qquad\quad 6\frac{5}{5} + \frac{3}{5} = 6\frac{8}{5}$

3. Now you have a different version of the original problem: $\qquad 6\frac{8}{5} - 2\frac{4}{5}$

4. Subtract the fractional parts of the two mixed numbers: $\qquad \frac{8}{5} - \frac{4}{5} = \frac{4}{5}$

5. Subtract the whole number parts of the two mixed numbers: $\qquad 6 - 2 = 4$

6. Add the results of the last 2 steps together: $\qquad\qquad\quad 4 + \frac{4}{5} = 4\frac{4}{5}$

Try these subtraction problems:

_____**14.** $\frac{4}{5} - \frac{2}{3}$

_____**15.** $\frac{7}{8} - \frac{1}{4} - \frac{1}{2}$

_____**16.** $4\frac{1}{3} - 2\frac{3}{4}$

Now let's put what you've learned about adding and subtracting fractions to work in some real-life problems.

_____**17.** Patrolman Peterson drove $3\frac{1}{2}$ miles to the police station. Then he drove $4\frac{3}{4}$ miles to his first assignment. When he left there, he drove 2 miles to his next assignment. Then he drove $3\frac{2}{3}$ miles back to the police station for a meeting. Finally, he drove $3\frac{1}{2}$ miles home. How many miles did he travel in total?

a. $17\frac{5}{12}$ b. $16\frac{5}{12}$ c. $15\frac{7}{12}$ d. $15\frac{5}{12}$ e. $13\frac{11}{12}$

_____**18.** Before leaving the fire station, Firefighter Sorensen noted that the mileage gauge on Engine 2 registered $4{,}357\frac{4}{10}$ miles. When he arrived at the scene of the fire, the mileage gauge then registered $4{,}400\frac{1}{10}$ miles. How many miles did he drive from the station to the fire scene?

a. $42\frac{3}{10}$ b. $42\frac{7}{10}$ c. $43\frac{7}{10}$ d. $47\frac{2}{10}$ e. $57\frac{3}{10}$

MULTIPLYING FRACTIONS

Multiplying fractions is actually easier than adding them. All you do is multiply the top numbers and then multiply the bottom numbers.

Examples: $\quad \frac{2}{3} \times \frac{5}{7} = \frac{2 \times 5}{3 \times 7} = \frac{10}{21} \qquad \frac{1}{2} \times \frac{3}{5} \times \frac{7}{4} = \frac{1 \times 3 \times 7}{2 \times 5 \times 4} = \frac{21}{40}$

Sometimes you can *cancel* before multiplying. Cancelling is a shortcut that makes the multiplication go faster because you're multiplying with smaller numbers. It's very similar to reducing: if there is a number that divides evenly into a top number and bottom number, do that division before multiplying. If you forget to cancel, you'll still get the right answer, but you'll have to reduce it.

Example: $\frac{5}{6} \times \frac{9}{20}$

1. Cancel the 6 and the 9 by dividing 3 into both of them: $6 \div 3 = 2$ and $9 \div 3 = 3$. Cross out the 6 and the 9.

$$\frac{5}{\overset{2}{\cancel{6}}} \times \frac{\overset{3}{\cancel{9}}}{20}$$

2. Cancel the 5 and the 20 by dividing 5 into both of them: $5 \div 5 = 1$ and $20 \div 5 = 4$. Cross out the 5 and the 20.

$$\frac{\overset{1}{\cancel{5}}}{\overset{2}{\cancel{6}}} \times \frac{\overset{3}{\cancel{9}}}{\underset{4}{\cancel{20}}}$$

3. Multiply across the new top numbers and the new bottom numbers:

$$\frac{1 \times 3}{2 \times 4} = \frac{3}{8}$$

Try these multiplication problems:

_____**19.** $\frac{1}{5} \times \frac{2}{3}$

_____**20.** $\frac{2}{3} \times \frac{4}{7} \times \frac{3}{5}$

_____**21.** $\frac{3}{4} \times \frac{8}{9}$

To multiply a fraction by a whole number, first rewrite the whole number as a fraction with a bottom number of 1:

Example: $5 \times \frac{2}{3} = \frac{5}{1} \times \frac{2}{3} = \frac{10}{3}$ (Optional: convert $\frac{10}{3}$ to a mixed number: $3\frac{1}{3}$)

To multiply with mixed numbers, it's easier to change them to improper fractions before multiplying.

Example: $4\frac{2}{3} \times 5\frac{1}{2}$

1. Convert $4\frac{2}{3}$ to an improper fraction: $4\frac{2}{3} = \frac{4 \times 3 + 2}{3} = \frac{14}{3}$

2. Convert $5\frac{1}{2}$ to an improper fraction: $5\frac{1}{2} = \frac{5 \times 2 + 1}{2} = \frac{11}{2}$

3. Cancel and multiply the fractions: $\frac{\overset{7}{\cancel{14}}}{3} \times \frac{11}{\underset{1}{\cancel{2}}} = \frac{77}{3}$

4. Optional: convert the improper fraction to a mixed number: $\frac{77}{3} = 25\frac{2}{3}$

Now try these multiplication problems with mixed numbers and whole numbers:

_____**22.** $4\frac{1}{3} \times \frac{2}{5}$

_____**23.** $2\frac{1}{2} \times 6$

_____**24.** $3\frac{3}{4} \times 4\frac{2}{5}$

Here are a few more real-life problems to test your skills:

_____**25.** After driving $\frac{2}{3}$ of the 15 miles to work, Mr. Stone stopped to make a phone call. How many miles had he driven when he made his call?
    a. 5   **b.** $7\frac{1}{2}$ **c.** 10   **d.** 12   **e.** $15\frac{2}{3}$

_____**26.** If Henry worked $\frac{3}{4}$ of a 40-hour week, how many hours did he work?
    a. $7\frac{1}{2}$ **b.** 10   **c.** 20   **d.** 25   **e.** 30

_____**27.** Technician Chin makes $14.00 an hour. When she works more than 8 hours a day, she gets overtime pay of $1\frac{1}{2}$ times her regular hourly wage for the extra hours. How much did she earn for working 11 hours in one day?
    a. $77   **b.** $154   **c.** $175   **d.** $210   **e.** $231

DIVIDING FRACTIONS

To divide one fraction by a second fraction, invert the second fraction (that is, flip the top and bottom numbers) and then multiply. That's all there is to it!

    Example: $\frac{1}{2} \div \frac{3}{5}$

1. Invert the second fraction ($\frac{3}{5}$): $\frac{5}{3}$

2. Change the division sign ($\div$) to a multiplication sign ($\times$)

3. Multiply the first fraction by the new second fraction: $\frac{1}{2} \times \frac{5}{3} = \frac{1 \times 5}{2 \times 3} = \frac{5}{6}$

To divide a fraction by a whole number, first change the whole number to a fraction by putting it over 1. Then follow the division steps above.

    Example: $\frac{3}{5} \div 2 = \frac{3}{5} \div \frac{2}{1} = \frac{3}{5} \times \frac{1}{2} = \frac{3 \times 1}{5 \times 2} = \frac{3}{10}$

When the division problem has a mixed number, convert it to an improper fraction and then divide as usual.

    Example: $2\frac{3}{4} \div \frac{1}{6}$

1. Convert $2\frac{3}{4}$ to an improper fraction: $2\frac{3}{4} = \frac{2 \times 4 + 3}{4} = \frac{11}{4}$

2. Divide $\frac{11}{4}$ by $\frac{1}{6}$: $\frac{11}{4} \div \frac{1}{6} = \frac{11}{4} \times \frac{6}{1}$

3. Flip $\frac{1}{6}$ to $\frac{6}{1}$, change $\div$ to $\times$, cancel and multiply: $\frac{11}{\underset{2}{4}} \times \frac{\overset{3}{6}}{1} = \frac{11 \times 3}{2 \times 1} = \frac{33}{2}$

Here are a few division problems to try:

_____**28.** $\frac{1}{3} \div \frac{2}{3}$

_____**29.** $2\frac{3}{4} \div \frac{1}{2}$

_____**30.** $\frac{3}{5} \div 3$

_____**31.** $3\frac{3}{4} \div 2\frac{1}{3}$

Let's wrap this up with some real-life problems.

_____**32.** If four friends evenly split $6\frac{1}{2}$ pounds of candy, how many pounds of candy does each friend get?
   a. $\frac{8}{13}$ b. $1\frac{5}{8}$ c. $1\frac{1}{2}$ d. $1\frac{5}{13}$ e. 4

_____**33.** How many $2\frac{1}{2}$-pound chunks of cheese can be cut from a single 20-pound piece of cheese?
   a. 2   b. 4   c. 6   d. 8   e. 10

_____**34.** Ms. Goldbaum earned $36.75 for working $3\frac{1}{2}$ hours. What was her hourly wage?
   a. $10.00   b. $10.50   c. $10.75   d. $12.00   e. $12.25

DECIMALS

WHAT IS A DECIMAL?

A decimal is a special kind of fraction. You use decimals every day when you deal with money—$10.35 is a decimal that represents 10 dollars and 35 cents. The decimal point separates the dollars from the cents. Because there are 100 cents in one dollar, 1¢ is $\frac{1}{100}$ of a dollar, or $.01.

Each decimal digit to the right of the decimal point has a name:

Example: $.1 = 1$ tenth $= \frac{1}{10}$
             $.02 = 2$ hundredths $= \frac{2}{100}$
             $.003 = 3$ thousandths $= \frac{3}{1000}$
             $.0004 = 4$ ten-thousandths $= \frac{4}{10,000}$

When you add zeroes after the rightmost decimal place, you don't change the value of the decimal. For example, 6.17 is the same as all of these:

6.170

6.1700

6.17000000000000000

If there are digits on both sides of the decimal point (like 10.35), the number is called a mixed decimal. If there are digits only to the right of the decimal point (like .53), the number is called a decimal. A whole number (like 15) is understood to have a decimal point at its right (15.). Thus, 15 is the same as 15.0, 15.00, 15.000, and so on.

CHANGING FRACTIONS TO DECIMALS

To change a fraction to a decimal, divide the bottom number into the top number after you put a decimal point and a few zeroes on the right of the top number. When you divide, bring the decimal point up into your answer.

Example: Change $\frac{3}{4}$ to a decimal.

1. Add a decimal point and 2 zeroes to the top number (3):   3.00
2. Divide the bottom number (4) into 3.00:

$$\begin{array}{r} .75 \\ 4\overline{)3.00} \\ \underline{2\,8} \\ 20 \\ \underline{20} \\ 0 \end{array}$$

   Bring the decimal point up into the answer:

3. The quotient (result of the division) is the answer: .75

Some fractions may require you to add many decimal zeroes in order for the division to come out evenly. In fact, when you convert a fraction like $\frac{2}{3}$ to a decimal, you can keep adding decimal zeroes to the top number forever because the division will never come out evenly! As you divide 3 into 2, you'll keep getting 6's:

$$2 \div 3 = .6666666666 \text{ etc}$$

This is called a *repeating decimal* and it can be written as $.66\overline{6}$ or as $.66\frac{2}{3}$. You can approximate it as .67, .667, .6667, and so on.

CHANGING DECIMALS TO FRACTIONS

To change a decimal to a fraction, write the digits of the decimal as the top number of a fraction and write the decimal's name as the bottom number of the fraction. Then reduce the fraction, if possible.

Example: .018

1. Write 18 as the top of the fraction: $\frac{18}{}$
2. Three places to the right of the decimal means *thousandths*, so write 1000 as the bottom number: $\frac{18}{1000}$
3. Reduce by dividing 2 into the top and bottom numbers: $\frac{18 \div 2}{1000 \div 2} = \frac{9}{500}$

Change these decimals or mixed decimals to fractions:

_____**35.** .005

_____**36.** 3.48

_____**37.** 123.456

COMPARING DECIMALS

Because decimals are easier to compare when they have the same number of digits after the decimal point, tack zeroes onto the end of the shorter decimals. Then all you have to do is compare the numbers as if the decimal points weren't there:

Example: Compare .08 and .1

1. Tack one zero at the end of .1:   .10
2. To compare .10 to .08, just compare 10 to 8.
3. Since 10 is larger than 8, .1 is larger than .08.

ADDING AND SUBTRACTING DECIMALS

To add or subtract decimals, line them up so their decimal points are even. You may want to tack on zeroes at the end of shorter decimals so you can keep all your digits lined up evenly. Remember, if a number doesn't have a decimal point, then put one at the right end of the number.

Example: 1.23 + 57 + .038

1. Line up the numbers like this:

$$
\begin{array}{r}
1.230 \\
57.000 \\
+\ \ .038 \\
\hline
\end{array}
$$

2. Add: 58.268

Example: 1.23 − .038

1. Line up the numbers like this:

$$
\begin{array}{r}
1.230 \\
-\ \ .038 \\
\hline
\end{array}
$$

2. Subtract: 1.192

Try these addition and subtraction problems:

_____**38.** .905 + .02 + 3.075

_____**39.** .005 + 8 + .3

_____**40.** 3.48 − 2.573

_____**41.** 123.456 − 122

_____**42.** Officer Peterson drove 3.7 miles to the state park. He then walked 1.6 miles around the park to make sure everything was all right. He got back into the car, drove 2.75 miles to check on a broken traffic light and then drove 2 miles back to the police station. How many miles did he drive in total?

a. 8.05   b. 8.45   c. 8.8   d. 10   e. 10.05

_____**43.** The average number of emergency room visits at City Hospital fell from 486.4 per week to 402.5 per week. By how many emergency room visits per week did the average fall?

a. 73.9   b. 83   c. 83.1   d. 83.9   e. 84.9

MULTIPLYING DECIMALS

To multiply decimals, ignore the decimal points and just multiply the numbers. Then count the total number of decimal digits (the digits to the *right* of the decimal point) in the numbers you're multiplying. Count off that number of digits in your answer beginning at the right side and put the decimal point to the *left* of those digits.

Example: 215.7×2.4

1. Multiply 2157 times 24:

$$
\begin{array}{r}
2157 \\
\times\ \ 24 \\
\hline
8628 \\
4314\ \ \\
\hline
51768 \\
\end{array}
$$

2. Because there are a total of 2 decimal digits in 215.7 and 2.4, count off 2 places from the right in 51768, placing the decimal point to the *left* of the last 2 digits:

517.68

If your answer doesn't have enough digits, tack zeroes on to the left of the answer.

Example: $.03 \times .006$

1. Multiply 3 times 6: $3 \times 6 = 18$

2. You need 5 decimal digits in your answer, so tack on 3 zeroes: 00018

3. Put the decimal point at the front of the number (which is 5 digits in from the right):   .00018

You can practice multiplying decimals with these:

_____**44.** $.05 \times .6$

_____**45.** $.053 \times 6.4$

_____**46.** $38.1 \times .0184$

_____**47.** Joe earns $14.50 per hour. Last week he worked 37.5 hours. How much money did he earn that week?

   a. $518.00   **b.** $518.50   **c.** $525.00   **d.** $536.50   **e.** $543.75

_____**48.** Nuts cost $3.50 per pound. Approximately how much will 4.25 pounds of nuts cost?

   a. $12.25   **b.** $12.50   **c.** $12.88   **d.** $14.50   **e.** $14.88

DIVIDING DECIMALS

To divide a decimal by a whole number, set up the division ($8\overline{).256}$) and immediately bring the decimal point straight up into the answer ($8\overline{).256}$). Then divide as you would normally divide whole numbers:

Example:

$$
\begin{array}{r}
.032 \\
8\overline{).256} \\
\underline{0} \\
25 \\
\underline{24} \\
16 \\
\underline{16} \\
0
\end{array}
$$

To divide any number by a decimal, there is an extra step to perform before you can divide. Move the decimal point to the very right of the number you're dividing by, counting the number of places you're moving it. Then move the decimal point the same number of places to the right in the number you're dividing into. In other words, first change the problem to one in which you're dividing by a whole number.

Example: $.06\overline{)1.218}$

1. Because there are 2 decimal digits in .06, move the decimal point 2 places to the right in both numbers and move the decimal point straight up into the answer:

$$.06.\overline{)1.21.8}$$

2. Divide using the new numbers:

$$
\begin{array}{r}
20.3 \\
6\overline{)121.8} \\
\underline{12} \\
01 \\
\underline{00} \\
18 \\
\underline{18} \\
0
\end{array}
$$

Under certain conditions, you have to tack on zeroes to the right of the last decimal digit in number you're dividing into:

- If there aren't enough digits for you to move the decimal point to the right, or
- If the answer doesn't come out evenly when you do the division, or
- If you're dividing a whole number by a decimal. Then you'll have to tack on the decimal point as well as some zeroes.

Try your skills on these division problems:

_____**49.** $7\overline{)9.8}$

_____**50.** $.0004\overline{).0512}$

_____**51.** $.05\overline{)28.6}$

_____**52.** $.14\overline{)196}$

_____**53.** If James Worthington drove his truck 92.4 miles in 2.1 hours, what was his average speed in miles per hour?

      a. 41   **b.** 44   **c.** 90.3   **d.** 94.5   **e.** 194.04

_____**54.** Mary Sanders walked a total of 18.6 miles in 4 days. On average, how many miles did she walk each day?

      a. 4.15   **b.** 4.60   **c.** 4.65   **d.** 22.60   **e.** 74.40

PERCENTS

WHAT IS A PERCENT?

A percent is a special kind of fraction or part of something. The bottom number (the *denominator*) is always 100. For example, 17% is the same as $\frac{17}{100}$. Literally, the word *percent* means *per 100 parts*. The root *cent* means 100: a *cent*ury is 100 years, there are 100 *cents* in a dollar, etc. Thus, 17% means 17 parts out of 100. Because fractions can also be expressed as decimals, 17% is also equivalent to .17, which is 17 hundredths.

You come into contact with percents every day. Sales tax, interest, and discounts are just a few common examples.

If you're shaky on fractions, you may want to review the fraction section before reading further.

CHANGING A DECIMAL TO A PERCENT AND VICE VERSA

To change a decimal to a percent, move the decimal point two places to the **right** and tack on a percent sign (%) at the end. If the decimal point moves to the very right of the number, you don't have to write the decimal point. If there aren't enough places to move the decimal point, add zeroes on the **right** before moving the decimal point.

To change a percent to a decimal, drop off the percent sign and move the decimal point two places to the **left**. If there aren't enough places to move the decimal point, add zeroes on the **left** before moving the decimal point.

Try changing these decimals to percents:

_____ **55.** .45

_____ **56.** .008

_____ **57.** .16$\frac{2}{3}$

Now change these percents to decimals:

_____ **58.** 12%

_____ **59.** 87$\frac{1}{2}$%

_____ **60.** 250%

CHANGING A FRACTION TO A PERCENT AND VICE VERSA

To change a fraction to a percent, there are two techniques. Each is illustrated by changing the fraction $\frac{1}{4}$ to a percent:

Technique 1: Multiply the fraction by 100%.

Multiply $\frac{1}{4}$ by 100%:

$$\frac{1}{\cancel{4}_1} \times \frac{\cancel{100}^{25}\%}{1} = 25\%$$

Technique 2: Divide the fraction's bottom number into the top number; then move the decimal point two places to the **right** and tack on a percent sign (%).

Divide 4 into 1 and move the decimal point 2 places to the right:

$$4\overline{)1.00}^{.25} \qquad .25 = 25\%$$

To change a percent to a fraction, remove the percent sign and write the number over 100. Then reduce if possible.

Example: Change 4% to a fraction

1. Remove the % and write the fraction 4 over 100: $\qquad \frac{4}{100}$

2. Reduce: $\qquad \frac{4 \div 4}{100 \div 4} = \frac{1}{25}$

Here's a more complicated example: Change 16$\frac{2}{3}$% to a fraction

1. Remove the % and write the fraction 16$\frac{2}{3}$ over 100: $\qquad \dfrac{16\frac{2}{3}}{100}$

2. Since a fraction means "top number divided by bottom number," rewrite the fraction as a division problem:

$16\frac{2}{3} \div 100$

3. Change the mixed number ($16\frac{2}{3}$) to an improper fraction ($\frac{50}{3}$):

$\frac{50}{3} \div \frac{100}{1}$

4. Flip the second fraction ($\frac{100}{1}$) and multiply:

$\frac{\overset{1}{50}}{3} \times \frac{1}{\underset{2}{100}} = \frac{1}{6}$

Try changing these fractions to percents:

_____ **61.** $\frac{1}{8}$

_____ **62.** $\frac{13}{25}$

_____ **63.** $\frac{7}{12}$

Now change these percents to fractions:

_____ **64.** 95%

_____ **65.** $37\frac{1}{2}$%

_____ **66.** 125%

Sometimes it is more convenient to work with a percentage as a fraction or a decimal. Rather than have to *calculate* the equivalent fraction or decimal, consider memorizing the equivalence table below. Not only will this increase your efficiency on the math test, but it will also be practical for real life situations.

CONVERSION TABLE

Decimal	%	Fraction
.25	25%	$\frac{1}{4}$
.50	50%	$\frac{1}{2}$
.75	75%	$\frac{3}{4}$
.10	10%	$\frac{1}{10}$
.20	20%	$\frac{1}{5}$
.40	40%	$\frac{2}{5}$
.60	60%	$\frac{3}{5}$
.80	80%	$\frac{4}{5}$
.33$\overline{3}$	$33\frac{1}{3}$%	$\frac{1}{3}$
.66$\overline{6}$	$66\frac{2}{3}$%	$\frac{2}{3}$

PERCENT WORD PROBLEMS

Word problems involving percents come in three main varieties:

- Find a percent of a whole.

  Example: What is 30% of 40?

- Find what percent one number is of another number.

  Example: 12 is what percent of 40?

- Find the whole when the percent of it is given.

  Example: 12 is 30% of what number?

While each variety has its own approach, there is a single shortcut formula you can use to solve each of these:

$$\frac{is}{of} = \frac{\%}{100}$$

The *is* is the number that usually follows or is just before the word *is* in the question.

The *of* is the number that usually follows the word *of* in the question.

The **%** is the number that in front of the **%** or *percent* in the question.

Or you may think of the shortcut formula as:

$$\frac{part}{whole} = \frac{\%}{100}$$

To solve each of the three varieties, we're going to use the fact that the **cross-products** are equal. The cross-products are the products of the numbers diagonally across from each other. Remembering that *product* means *multiply*, here's how to create the cross-products for the percent shortcut:

$$\frac{part}{whole} = \frac{\%}{100}$$
$$part \times 100 = whole \times \%$$

Here's how to use the shortcut with cross-products:

- Find a percent of a whole.

  What is 30% of 40?

  30 is the % and 40 is the *of* number:

  Cross-multiply and solve for *is*:

  $$\frac{is}{40} = \frac{30}{100}$$
  $$is \times 100 = 40 \times 30$$
  $$is \times 100 = 1200$$
  $$12 \times 100 = 1200$$

  Thus, **12** *is* 30% of 40.

- Find what percent one number is of another number.

  12 is what percent of 40?

  12 is the *is* number and 40 is the *of* number:

  Cross-multiply and solve for %:

  $$\frac{12}{40} = \frac{\%}{100}$$
  $$12 \times 100 = 40 \times \%$$
  $$1200 = 40 \times \%$$
  $$1200 = 40 \times \mathbf{30}$$

  Thus, 12 is **30%** of 40.

■ Find the whole when the percent of it is given.

12 is 30% of what number?

12 is the *is* number and 30 is the *%*:
$$\frac{12}{of} = \frac{30}{100}$$

Cross-multiply and solve for the *of* number:
$$12 \times 100 = of \times 30$$
$$1200 = of \times 30$$
$$1200 = \mathbf{40} \times 30$$

Thus 12 is 30% *of* 40.

You can use the same technique to find the percent increase or decrease. The *is* number is the actual increase or decrease, and the *of* number is the original amount.

Example: If a merchant puts his $20 hats on sale for $15, by what percent does he decrease the selling price?

1. Calculate the decrease, the *is* number: $20 − $15 = $5

2. The *of* number is the original amount, $20

3. Set up the equation and solve for *of* by cross-multiplying:
$$\frac{5}{20} = \frac{\%}{100}$$
$$5 \times 100 = 20 \times \%$$
$$500 = 20 \times \%$$
$$500 = 20 \times \mathbf{25}$$

4. Thus, the selling price is decreased by **25%**.

If the merchant later raises the price of the hats from $15 back to $20, don't be fooled into thinking that the percent increase is also 25%! It's actually more, because the increase amount of $5 is now based on a lower original price of only $15:
$$\frac{5}{15} = \frac{\%}{100}$$
$$5 \times 100 = 15 \times \%$$
$$500 = 15 \times \%$$
$$500 = 15 \times 33\tfrac{1}{3}$$

Thus, the selling price is increased by **33%**.

Find a percent of a whole:

_____**67.** 1% of 25

_____**68.** 18.2% of 50

_____**69.** $37\tfrac{1}{2}$% of 100

_____**70.** 125% of 60

Find what percent one number is of another number.

_____**71.** 10 is what % of 20?

_____**72.** 4 is what % of 12?

_____**73.** 12 is what % of 4?

Find the whole when the percent of it is given.

_____**74.** 15% of what number is 15?

_____**75.** $37\frac{1}{2}$% of what number is 3?

_____**76.** 200% of what number is 20?

Now try your percent skills on some real life problems.

_____**77.** Last Monday, 20% of the 140-member nursing staff was absent. How many nurses were absent that day?
a. 14   b. 20   c. 28   d. 112   e. 126

_____**78.** 40% of Vero's postal service employees are women. If there are 80 women in Vero's postal service, how many men are employed there?
a. 32   b. 112   c. 120   d. 160   e. 200

_____**79.** Of the 840 crimes committed last month, 42 involved petty theft. What percent of the crimes involved petty theft?
a. .5%   b. 2%   c. 5%   d. 20%   e. 50%

_____**80.** Sam's Shoe Store put all of its merchandise on sale for 20% off. If Jason saved $10 by purchasing one pair of shoes during the sale, what was the original price of the shoes before the sale?
a. $12   b. $20   c. $40   d. $50   e. $70

ROBLEMS

28. $\frac{1}{2}$

29. $5\frac{1}{2}$

30. $\frac{1}{5}$

31. $\frac{45}{28}$ or $1\frac{17}{28}$

32. b

33. d

34. b

DECIMALS

35. $\frac{5}{1000}$ or $\frac{1}{200}$

36. $3\frac{12}{25}$

37. $123\frac{456}{1000}$ or $123\frac{57}{125}$

38. 4

39. 8.305

40. .907

41. 1.456

42. b

43. d

44. .03

45. .3392

46. .70104

47. e

48. e

49. 1.4

50. 128

51. 572

52. 1400

53. b

54. c

PERCENTS

55. 45%

56. .8%

57. 16.67% or $16\frac{2}{3}$%

58. .12

59. .875

60. 2.5

61. 12.5% or $12\frac{1}{2}$%

62. 52%

63. 58.33% or $58\frac{1}{3}$%

64. $\frac{19}{20}$

65. $\frac{3}{8}$

66. $\frac{5}{4}$ or $1\frac{1}{4}$

67. $\frac{1}{4}$ or .25

68. 9.1

69. $37\frac{1}{2}$ or 37.5

70. 75

71. 50%

72. $33\frac{1}{3}$%

73. 300%

74. 100

75. 8

76. 10

77. c

78. c

79. c

80. d

12. $\frac{55}{24}$ or $2\frac{7}{24}$

13. $7\frac{1}{4}$

14. $\frac{2}{15}$

15. $\frac{1}{8}$

16. $\frac{19}{12}$ or $1\frac{7}{12}$

17. a

18. b

19. $\frac{2}{15}$

20. $\frac{8}{35}$

21. $\frac{2}{3}$

22. $\frac{26}{15}$ or $1\frac{11}{15}$

23. 15

24. $\frac{33}{2}$ or $16\frac{1}{2}$

25. c

26. e

27. c

SANITATION WORKER PRACTICE EXAM 2

11

CHAPTER SUMMARY

This is the second of three practice exams in this book based on Sanitation Worker exams given in various cities around the U.S.. After working through the instructional material in the previous chapters, take this test to see how much your score has improved since you took the first exam.

The exam that follows is based on the areas most commonly tested on written exams for the position of sanitation worker. Though your exam may differ somewhat from the exam you're about to take, you are likely to find that most of the same skills are tested on the exam in your city. This test includes 70 multiple-choice questions on understanding written language, communicating information, using judgment to recognize a problem, following rules, using spatial reasoning, and math.

For this exam, simulate the actual test-taking experience as much as possible. Find a quiet place to work where you won't be interrupted. Tear out the answer sheet on the next page and find some number 2 pencils to fill in the circles with. Set a timer or stopwatch, and give yourself two hours for the entire exam.

After the exam, use the answer key that follows it to see how you did and to find out why the correct answers are correct. The answer key is followed by a section on how to score your exam.

1.	ⓐ	ⓑ	ⓒ	ⓓ		25.	ⓐ	ⓑ	ⓒ	ⓓ		49.	ⓐ	ⓑ	ⓒ	ⓓ
2.	ⓐ	ⓑ	ⓒ	ⓓ		26.	ⓐ	ⓑ	ⓒ	ⓓ		50.	ⓐ	ⓑ	ⓒ	ⓓ
3.	ⓐ	ⓑ	ⓒ	ⓓ		27.	ⓐ	ⓑ	ⓒ	ⓓ		51.	ⓐ	ⓑ	ⓒ	ⓓ
4.	ⓐ	ⓑ	ⓒ	ⓓ		28.	ⓐ	ⓑ	ⓒ	ⓓ		52.	ⓐ	ⓑ	ⓒ	ⓓ
5.	ⓐ	ⓑ	ⓒ	ⓓ		29.	ⓐ	ⓑ	ⓒ	ⓓ		53.	ⓐ	ⓑ	ⓒ	ⓓ
6.	ⓐ	ⓑ	ⓒ	ⓓ		30.	ⓐ	ⓑ	ⓒ	ⓓ		54.	ⓐ	ⓑ	ⓒ	ⓓ
7.	ⓐ	ⓑ	ⓒ	ⓓ		31.	ⓐ	ⓑ	ⓒ	ⓓ		55.	ⓐ	ⓑ	ⓒ	ⓓ
8.	ⓐ	ⓑ	ⓒ	ⓓ		32.	ⓐ	ⓑ	ⓒ	ⓓ		56.	ⓐ	ⓑ	ⓒ	ⓓ
9.	ⓐ	ⓑ	ⓒ	ⓓ		33.	ⓐ	ⓑ	ⓒ	ⓓ		57.	ⓐ	ⓑ	ⓒ	ⓓ
10.	ⓐ	ⓑ	ⓒ	ⓓ		34.	ⓐ	ⓑ	ⓒ	ⓓ		58.	ⓐ	ⓑ	ⓒ	ⓓ
11.	ⓐ	ⓑ	ⓒ	ⓓ		35.	ⓐ	ⓑ	ⓒ	ⓓ		59.	ⓐ	ⓑ	ⓒ	ⓓ
12.	ⓐ	ⓑ	ⓒ	ⓓ		36.	ⓐ	ⓑ	ⓒ	ⓓ		60.	ⓐ	ⓑ	ⓒ	ⓓ
13.	ⓐ	ⓑ	ⓒ	ⓓ		37.	ⓐ	ⓑ	ⓒ	ⓓ		61.	ⓐ	ⓑ	ⓒ	ⓓ
14.	ⓐ	ⓑ	ⓒ	ⓓ		38.	ⓐ	ⓑ	ⓒ	ⓓ		62.	ⓐ	ⓑ	ⓒ	ⓓ
15.	ⓐ	ⓑ	ⓒ	ⓓ		39.	ⓐ	ⓑ	ⓒ	ⓓ		63.	ⓐ	ⓑ	ⓒ	ⓓ
16.	ⓐ	ⓑ	ⓒ	ⓓ		40.	ⓐ	ⓑ	ⓒ	ⓓ		64.	ⓐ	ⓑ	ⓒ	ⓓ
17.	ⓐ	ⓑ	ⓒ	ⓓ		41.	ⓐ	ⓑ	ⓒ	ⓓ		65.	ⓐ	ⓑ	ⓒ	ⓓ
18.	ⓐ	ⓑ	ⓒ	ⓓ		42.	ⓐ	ⓑ	ⓒ	ⓓ		66.	ⓐ	ⓑ	ⓒ	ⓓ
19.	ⓐ	ⓑ	ⓒ	ⓓ		43.	ⓐ	ⓑ	ⓒ	ⓓ		67.	ⓐ	ⓑ	ⓒ	ⓓ
20.	ⓐ	ⓑ	ⓒ	ⓓ		44.	ⓐ	ⓑ	ⓒ	ⓓ		68.	ⓐ	ⓑ	ⓒ	ⓓ
21.	ⓐ	ⓑ	ⓒ	ⓓ		45.	ⓐ	ⓑ	ⓒ	ⓓ		69.	ⓐ	ⓑ	ⓒ	ⓓ
22.	ⓐ	ⓑ	ⓒ	ⓓ		46.	ⓐ	ⓑ	ⓒ	ⓓ		70.	ⓐ	ⓑ	ⓒ	ⓓ
23.	ⓐ	ⓑ	ⓒ	ⓓ		47.	ⓐ	ⓑ	ⓒ	ⓓ						
24.	ⓐ	ⓑ	ⓒ	ⓓ		48.	ⓐ	ⓑ	ⓒ	ⓓ						

SANITATION WORKER EXAM 2

Answer questions 1–3 on the basis of the following information.

Beginning next month, the Sanitation Department will institute a program intended to remove the graffiti from sanitation trucks. Any truck that finishes its assigned route before the end of the workers' shift will return to the sanitation lot, where supervisors will provide materials for workers to use in cleaning the trucks. Because the length of time it takes to complete different routes varies, trucks will no longer be assigned to a specific route but will be rotated among the routes. Therefore, workers should no longer leave personal items in the trucks, as they will not necessarily be using the same truck each day as they did in the past.

1. According to the passage, the removal of graffiti from sanitation trucks will be done by
   a. sanitation supervisors
   b. sanitation workers
   c. custodial staff
   d. persons who created the graffiti

2. According to the passage, which of the following is true of sanitation routes?
   a. They are assigned according to the amount of graffiti on the truck in question.
   b. They are all of equal length, though some may take longer to drive than others.
   c. They take longer to complete at certain times of the year.
   d. They vary in the amount of time they take to complete.

3. According to the passage, prior to instituting the graffiti clean-up program, sanitation workers
   a. were not responsible for the condition of the trucks they drove
   b. had to repaint the trucks at regular intervals to get rid of graffiti
   c. usually drove or rode the same truck each work day
   d. were not allowed to leave personal belongings in the trucks

4. As you are driving your collection truck, you notice that the gas pedal is sticking. You shift the truck into neutral and then work the pedal back and forth to see if you can fix the problem. The pedal is still sticking but not as much as before. What should you do?
   a. continue on your route, relying on your brakes to stop you if the accelerator sticks again
   b. take the truck to the nearest mechanic and have the problem fixed
   c. call your supervisor to report a problem with your truck
   d. get out your tools and try to fix the problem

5. You wake up one morning with what feels like stomach flu. It is almost time to go to work. What should you do?
   a. force yourself to go to work for at least an hour or two and then leave work sick
   b. call in sick
   c. go to work and "tough out" the day
   d. get someone else to call in, so your supervisor will know you are really sick

6. While Sanitation Workers Halliday and Schmidt are making a pickup in front of the apartment building at 8870 Paris Road, Schmidt is cut on the hand by a large piece of broken glass. The glass had been carelessly placed in an unmarked plastic garbage bag. Because the cut requires stitches, Halliday drives Schmidt to City Hospital's emergency room two blocks away. While Schmidt receives medical care, Halliday phones his supervisor. Which of the following reports should Halliday give to describe the situation most clearly and accurately?

   a. Schmidt was cut on the hand by broken glass when we were collecting on Paris Road. We are at City Hospital where a doctor is stitching the cut.

   b. I drove Schmidt to the hospital because of the glass left on Paris Road, which is two blocks from where we were making our pickup.

   c. Schmidt cut his hand. I drove him to the emergency room after he had picked up a plastic bag and will receive stitches for the cut.

   d. There was broken glass at 8870 Paris Road where Schmidt required stitches at the emergency room at City Hospital. I drove him here.

Answer questions 7 and 8 on the basis of the following information.

AVERAGE NUMBER OF TONS OF GARBAGE COLLECTED

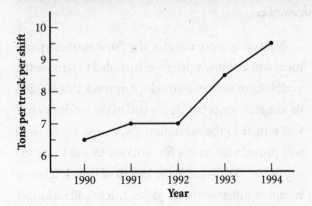

7. According to the graph, what was the number of tons of garbage collected per shift per truck in 1990?

   a. $6\frac{1}{2}$

   b. $7\frac{1}{2}$

   c. $8\frac{1}{2}$

   d. $9\frac{1}{2}$

8. According to the graph, which period of time showed the smallest increase in tons per truck per shift collected?

   a. 1990–1991

   b. 1991–1992

   c. 1992–1993

   d. 1993–1994

9. If it takes four sanitation workers 1 hour and 45 minutes to perform a particular job, how long would it take one sanitation worker to perform the same task alone?

   a. 4.5 hours

   b. 5 hours

   c. 7 hours

   d. 7.5 hours

10. If the average person throws away 3.5 pounds of trash every day, how much trash would the average person throw away in one week?
   a. 24.5 pounds
   b. 31.5 pounds
   c. 40.2 pounds
   d. 240 pounds

Answer questions 11–13 on the basis of the following information.

Next week the city will begin testing automated garbage collection trucks on a few routes. These trucks require only a driver, as the hydraulic arm lifts the garbage containers and empties them into the truck. Supervisors have been trained in operating the automated trucks and, for the next six months, one supervisor and two sanitation workers will ride in the trucks, so that the supervisors can train the workers. No worker may operate these trucks without three shifts of training. Sanitation workers will be assigned to the trucks on a rotating basis.

11. Which of the following can be inferred from the passage about the automated trucks?
   a. Only supervisors will ever be allowed to operate the automated trucks.
   b. Automated trucks are less dangerous than regular trucks.
   c. Sanitation workers will receive three shifts of training on the trucks in the next six months.
   d. Sanitation workers will train on the new trucks based on seniority.

12. According to the passage, automated garbage collection trucks
   a. require special training to operate
   b. are more expensive than regular garbage collection trucks

c. will never replace regular garbage collection trucks
d. are easier to operate than the old garbage collection trucks

13. During the next six months, all sanitation workers can expect to
   a. be replaced by automation
   b. be permanently assigned to the automated trucks
   c. train their coworkers in operation of the new trucks
   d. receive three shifts of training if assigned to one of the new trucks

Answer questions 14–16 based on the information in the following procedure.

Sanitation Department policy states that sanitation workers who witness an emergency situation are required to call for assistance. Workers are not expected to put themselves in danger but are expected to act responsibly in such a situation.

14. One icy afternoon while Sanitation Worker Lightsey is spreading salt on a busy street, a speeding vehicle slides into the intersection and crashes into a school bus. The damage seems minor. The school bus driver gets out and starts yelling at the person who was driving the car. What should Lightsey do?
   a. keep working, as the school bus driver is handling the situation
   b. call in the accident on the collection truck radio
   c. pull over near the bus and see if help is needed for any injured passengers
   d. spread salt around the accident site and then return to regular duties

15. Sanitation Worker Upton is collecting garbage at an apartment building when, from above, there comes a scream and a crashing noise. A second story balcony has given way on the building and a woman who had been standing on it has fallen. Upton tries to call on the truck radio for help but the radio won't transmit. What should Upton do?

a. go back to work, as any other action would put Upton in danger

b. find a phone or emergency call box and call from there

c. try to fix the radio and, if successful, call in the accident

d. look for the building superintendent to handle the situation

16. One winter afternoon in below-freezing weather, Sanitation Worker Jessup is emptying a wire basket at a busy downtown intersection. A nearby fire hydrant bursts suddenly, and water starts pouring out onto the street. What should Jessup do?

a. go for a salt truck because the water is going to freeze immediately

b. keep working because this is not an emergency situation

c. find a phone and call the fire department

d. call a supervisor on the radio for instructions on how to handle the problem

Answer questions 17–19 solely on the basis of the map on the facing page. The arrows indicate traffic flow; one arrow indicates a one-way street going in the direction of the arrow; two arrows represent a two-way street. You are not allowed to go the wrong way on a one-way street.

17. Sanitation Workers Moynahan and Chance have just finished lunch at Al's Cafe, which faces Jones Road. Their next garbage pick-up is at the Cleveland Avenue entrance to the Armbray Towers. What is their most direct legal route to the Armbray Towers?

a. go east on Jones Road, then south on Kennedy Boulevard, then west on Glade Road, and then north on Cleveland Avenue to the Armbray Towers

b. go west on Jones Road to Cleveland Avenue and then north on Cleveland to the Armbray Towers

c. go west on Jones Road, then south on Ford Road, then west on Glade Road, and then north on Cleveland Avenue to the Armbray Towers

d. go west on Jones Road, then north on Ford Road, then west on Palmer Road, then south on Taft Road, then west on Jones Road, and then north on Cleveland Avenue to the Armbray Towers

18. Sanitation Workers Moy and Packer are north-bound on Lincoln Street and have just crossed Alpen Street. They are headed to their first pick-up on Adams Avenue at Pine Avenue. What is their most direct legal route?

a. continue north on Lincoln Street, and then go east on Wilshire Avenue, then south on Ford Road, then east on Glade Road, and then south on Adams Avenue to Pine Avenue

b. continue north on Lincoln Street, and then go west on Palmer Road, then south on Taft Road, and then east on Pine Avenue to Adams Avenue

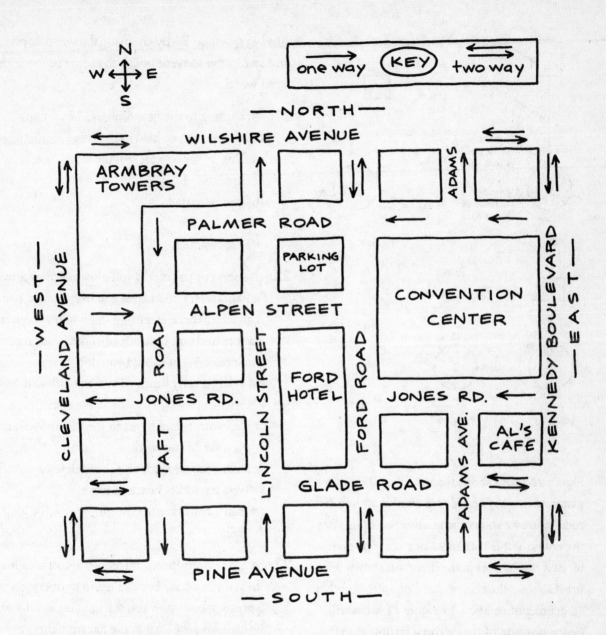

c. make a U-turn on Lincoln Street, and then go south on Lincoln Street and then east on Pine Avenue to Adams Avenue

d. continue north on Lincoln Street, and then go west on Wilshire Avenue, then south on Cleveland Avenue, and then east on Pine Avenue to Adams Avenue

19. Sanitation Worker Tonka is southbound on Kennedy Boulevard. He makes a right turn onto Glade Road, then a left onto Taft Road, then a right onto Pine Avenue and another right onto Cleveland Avenue, and then a right onto Wilshire Avenue. Which direction is he facing?

a. west

b. south

c. east

d. north

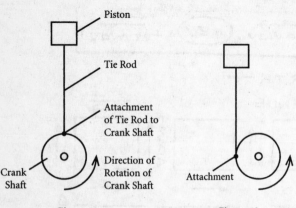

Figure #1

Figure #2

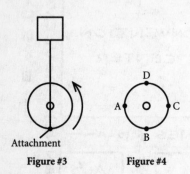

Figure #3   Figure #4

20. Figure #1 above shows the initial position of a piston that is connected to a crankshaft by a tie rod. Figure #2 shows the relative positions after the crankshaft is rotated 90 degrees (one quarter of a revolution) in the direction shown. Figure #3 shows the relative positions after another 90 degrees of rotation. In Figure #4, what will be the position of the tie rod attachment to the crankshaft after yet another 90 degree rotation?
  a. position A
  b. position B
  c. position C
  d. position D

Answer question 21 by choosing the word or phrase that means the same or nearly the same as the underlined word.

21. According to the new directive, "Every city employee will be held personally <u>accountable</u> for his or her conduct on the job."
  a. applauded
  b. compensated
  c. responsible
  d. approached

22. A friend of yours sees you plowing snow along a main artery and waves you over to talk. You can tell that she is settling in for a long conversation, and you have already taken your morning break. What should you do?
  a. take an early lunch so you can talk with your friend
  b. tell your friend to get in the cab and talk to you while you work
  c. talk a few seconds and then tell your friend you have to get back to work
  d. call a coworker to cover for you while you talk

23. It is noon, and snow mixed with sleet is falling heavily. You have been called in to operate a salt spreader, but when you start to check out your vehicle you notice that the hazard lights are not working. What should you do?
  a. tell your supervisor about the problem and say that you need a different spreader
  b. start your route, since you probably won't need hazard lights in the daytime
  c. start your route and then call for advice from the dispatcher
  d. stop by an auto parts store and buy new bulbs for the lights

24. Very early Monday morning, as Sanitation Worker Chang is driving on Roberts Road between Sheridan and Partridge Streets, he notices thick gray smoke coming from the front window of an insurance office that is located in the middle of the block. He parks the truck, runs up to the coffee shop two doors from the insurance office, and calls 911. Which of the following statements would most accurately describe the situation to the 911 operator?

a. I'm at the coffee shop on Roberts Road, and I can see smoke coming out of the window, which is between Sheridan and Partridge Streets. The insurance office is in the middle of the block.

b. There is thick smoke coming from the insurance office on Roberts Road. This office is in the middle of the block between Sheridan and Partridge Streets.

c. The insurance office where there is smoke is located in the middle of the block on Roberts Road and Partridge Street.

d. Two doors from the coffee shop in the middle of the block on Roberts Road there is thick smoke coming from the front window.

25. Junk cars are one of the most common complaints made by city residents to the Public Works Department. Sanitation Worker Martone notices the same car three weeks in a row in front of the building at 278 Glendale Avenue. He notes that it is an older model Chevrolet, very rusted and with one tire missing. The license number is RTH-450. Which of following reports should Martone give to describe the situation most clearly and accurately?

a. A rusted car three weeks old is sitting on Glendale Avenue with a license RTH-450 and a tire missing.

b. The car is a Chevrolet, 450-RTH, parked in front of 278 Glendale Avenue, which is very rusted and has one tire missing. It is probably a junk car.

c. There is a junk car, an older, rusted Chevrolet with the license RTH-450, sitting in front of the building at 278 Glendale. I first noticed it three weeks ago.

d. For three weeks at 278 Glendale Avenue, someone has been parking a car in front of the building. This is a rusted Chevrolet but the license is still there.

Answer questions 26 and 27 based on the following information.

All collisions involving Sanitation Department vehicles on Sanitation Department property must be reported immediately to supervisory staff. Sanitation workers are expected to call for medical attention first if the situation calls for it before asking for a supervisor.

26. Sanitation Worker Gonzales has checked out a collection truck and is backing the vehicle out of a parking slot without assistance. He backs into Sanitation Worker Erickson's salt spreader, crumpling the passenger side of that vehicle. What should Gonzales do now?

a. make sure Erickson is not hurt and then call for a supervisor

b. call for a supervisor and then check on Erickson and the salt spreader

c. arrange with Erickson to meet here at the end of the shift to report the accident

d. try to fix the damage himself without reporting the incident

27. Sanitation Worker Kare is looking down at her paperwork while driving at an ice and snow dump site. She runs into the back of another Sanitation Department vehicle and breaks her nose against the steering wheel. The other driver is not hurt. What should she do?
   a. call for a mechanic and then go to the hospital
   b. call for a supervisor and then call for an ambulance
   c. get a coworker to drive her to the hospital
   d. call for an ambulance and then call for a supervisor

Answer question 28 using the following calendar.

JUNE						
S	M	T	W	T	F	S
			1	2	3	4
5	6	7	8	9	10	11
12	13	14	15	16	17	18
19	20	21	22	23	24	25
26	27	28	29	30		

28. The City picks up recyclable materials only every other week. Using the calendar above, if a household has its recyclable items picked up on Wednesday, June 8, when can they expect the next pick up of recyclable items?
   a. June 15
   b. June 22
   c. June 29
   d. June 21

Answer question 29 by choosing the word or phrase that means the same or nearly the same as the underlined word.

29. Customer complaints must be handled in a <u>diplomatic</u> manner.
   a. tactful
   b. delaying
   c. elaborate
   d. combative

30. A five-year-old child walks up to you one afternoon as you are picking up trash on a residential street. He is crying and tells you that he is lost. What should you do?
   a. put him in the cab of your truck and let him ride with you until he's calm enough to remember where he lives
   b. call in using your truck radio and ask the dispatcher to send police to your location
   c. walk door-to-door with the boy until you find out which house is his
   d. take the boy to the nearest house and ask the residents to call the police and to take care of the boy till the police arrive

31. At the curb in front of an apartment building you see a sack of garbage, a torn bean bag chair, a plastic pickle barrel, and a wooden box. Which of these items will be easiest to roll to your truck?
   a. sack of garbage
   b. bean bag chair
   c. pickle barrel
   d. wooden box

32. The rain from last night has frozen, and you are operating a salt spreader. You see a sign just before you get to a bridge. The sign reads "Bridge Freezes Before Roadway." What should you do?
   a. speed up to get over the bridge before your tires slide

b. drive slowly while spreading the salt in case the bridge has ice on it

c. park the truck at the side of the road and wait for assistance

d. pump the brakes as you drive over the bridge in order to avoid a skid

33. The city collects bulky waste items on an appointment-only basis. Bulky waste is any item that will not fit in a 35-gallon can or bag. The charge for a pickup of bulky waste is $10.00 for the first item and $5.00 for each additional item. A householder stops Sanitation Worker Johnston to ask him why he did not pick up the old TV set that is sitting next to her garbage can. Which of the following statements best explains the city's bulky waste policy?

a. Bulky waste items left next to garbage cans will not be picked up unless there is an appointment. The fee is either $10.00 or $5.00.

b. For a charge of $10.00 for one item and $5.00 for two or more items, the city will pick up bulky waste items, which are items that will not fit into a 35-gallon bag or can. An appointment is necessary.

c. Bulky waste items which do not fit into a 35-gallon bag or can are collected only with an additional fee. The charge is on an appointment-basis only and costs $10.00 for the first item and $5.00 for the others.

d. Waste items that will not fit into a 35-gallon can or bag are collected by the city on an appointment-only basis. There is a $10.00 charge for one item; for each additional item, there is a $5.00 charge.

34. Sanitation Worker Banks is collecting garbage at 635 Dennison Road when he sees a late model red Camaro sideswipe a white Taurus that is parked across the street. When the driver of the Camaro does not stop, Banks tries to get the license number. He is able to read only the first two letters, which are WR. The resident at 635 Dennison also witnesses the accident and phones the police. Which of the following statements would Banks make to describe the incident most clearly and accurately when the police arrive?

a. As I was collecting garbage at 635 Dennison, I saw a red Camaro sideswipe the Taurus. When the driver of the Camaro didn't stop, I tried to get his license number. The first two letters are WR.

b. The car across the street on Dennison was sideswiped as I was collecting garbage, but I got part of the license. It's the white Taurus. The driver of the car didn't stop, which is how I only got the first two letters.

c. There was a red Camaro and the driver didn't want to stop on Dennison, so I checked his license, which contained a W and an R. The resident at 635 Dennison can tell you the details I didn't have.

d. While collecting garbage, a red Camaro was coming the other way at 635 Dennison. The Taurus got hit but he didn't stop. I was able to only read the W and R.

35. A sanitation worker knows that the floor of a large storage room has a width of 40 feet and a length of 42 feet. What is the area of that floor space?

a. 162 square feet

b. 168 square feet

c. 1,608 square feet

d. 1,680 square feet

36. Which of the following rope lengths is longest?
(1 cm = 0.39 inches)
a. 1 meter
b. 1 yard
c. 32 inches
d. 85 centimeters

37. You are driving a street sweeper and find a car illegally parked in your way. You've noticed this car illegally parked before. What should you do?
a. knock on apartment doors until you find the car's owner
b. carefully push the car out of the way with the sweeper
c. call your supervisor and ask for instructions
d. sweep around the car

38. You are collecting in a commercial district. As you are lifting a sack of garbage into the truck, the sack splits open and garbage falls into the street. What should you do?
a. sweep it into the gutter and let the street sweeper handle it
b. pick it up and put it in the truck
c. let the business that put it out clean it up, since the garbage probably wasn't packaged properly
d. go inside the business involved and ask for help cleaning up the mess

Answer questions 39–41 on the basis of the following information.

Sanitation workers are responsible for refueling their trucks at the end of each shift. All other routine maintenance is performed by maintenance department personnel, who are also responsible for maintaining service records. If a worker believes a truck is in need of mechanical repair, she or he should fill out the pink repair requisition form and turn it in to the shift supervisor. The worker should also notify the shift supervisor verbally whether, in the worker's opinion, the truck must be repaired immediately or may be driven for the rest of the shift.

39. If a truck is due to have the oil changed, this procedure will be done by
a. maintenance department personnel
b. sanitation workers
c. shift supervisors
d. outside contractors

40. The passage implies that sanitation trucks
a. are refueled when they have less than half a tank of gas
b. have the oil changed every 1,000 miles
c. are refueled at the end of every shift
d. are in frequent need of repair

41. Sanitation Worker Weston notices the truck that she is driving makes a grinding noise whenever it makes a left turn. Based on the passage, what is the first thing she should do?
a. call maintenance to repair the truck
b. return to the lot and exchange her truck for another
c. immediately stop at a phone and call the shift supervisor
d. fill out a repair requisition form and turn it in to the shift supervisor

42. You and your partner are collecting garbage on a city street. You realize that you will have to back the truck up about ten feet to get around a bus that has broken down, but you can't see what's behind your truck. What should you do?
a. wait until the problem with the bus is solved and then drive forward

b. help the bus driver push the bus out of the way

c. back up slowly and carefully, using your mirrors as much as possible

d. have your partner get out and guide you as you back up the truck

43. If a sanitation worker weighs 168 pounds, what is the approximate weight of that worker in kilograms? (1 kilogram = about 2.2 pounds)

a. 76

b. 87

c. 149

d. 150

44. Last year 220 city residents were cited for violating a local ordinance against open burning. Of those residents, 60% were fined for the violation. How many residents who violated the ordinance were not fined?

a. 36

b. 55

c. 88

d. 132

45. The Department of Streets and Sanitation is responsible for keeping the city's streets free of ice and snow during the winter months. Among these streets are 90 miles of priority snow routes, where parking is restricted every day from 2 a.m. to 6:30 a.m. between December 1 and March 31. Which of the following statements reports this policy most clearly and accurately?

a. There are 90 miles of snow routes in the city where parking is restricted all of December and March.

b. Between December 1 and March 31, parking is restricted every day from 2 a.m. to 6:30

a.m. on any street that is a priority snow route.

c. From December 1 until March 31, the city must keep all streets free of snow. Therefore, 90 miles of snow routes have been established from 2 a.m. to 6:30 a.m. each day.

d. Parking is restricted along priority snow routes from 2 a.m. to 6:30 a.m. until March 31 of each year for the purpose of keeping the city's streets clear.

46. While on your route early one morning, you find a human body stuffed into a garbage container. What should you do?

a. empty the container into the truck and drive straight to the police department

b. without moving the body, see if there is identification on it, and then call the police

c. put on your gloves, pull the body out of the container, and then call police

d. do not touch anything and use the truck radio to ask the dispatcher to call the police

47. Your partner shows up to work one morning intoxicated. He tells you he's been out all night drinking. He climbs behind the wheel of the garbage truck and insists on driving. What should you do?

a. take the keys from him and notify a supervisor

b. tell him you'll drive so he can sleep it off

c. call someone from his family to come and get him

d. tell him you'll drive but he has to pull his weight or you'll report him

48. Sanitation Worker Lindsay is on a new route. When he finishes collecting on Elm Street, he makes a right turn onto Beacon Avenue, not noticing that he is now going the wrong way on a one-way street. Before he realizes his mistake, a Toyota driven by Mary Gardner hits the front fender of Lindsay's truck. Neither driver is injured, but Mary Gardner's Toyota sustains considerable damage. Lindsay phones the police and his supervisor. Which of the following reports describes the incident most clearly and accurately?

    a. A car ran into me as I was making a right turn onto Beacon Avenue. The car is wrecked, but Mary Gardner is fine. It was a one-way street but I didn't know.

    b. A Toyota hit my truck, but it was my fault when I left Elm Street, which is one-way. Fortunately, there were no injuries.

    c. My truck was hit by a woman driving a Toyota. The accident was my fault because I was driving the wrong way on Beacon Avenue. No one is hurt but the Toyota is damaged.

    d. I hit a Toyota driving the wrong way on Beacon Avenue, a one-way street. Her car has been damaged but she has not.

49. Of the 1,125 employees in the Department of Public Works, 135 speak fluent Spanish. What percentage of the Public Works employees speaks fluent Spanish?

    a. 7.3%

    b. 8.3%

    c. 12%

    d. 14%

50. Workers on snow crews have to buy duty boots at the full price of $84.50, but workers who have served at least a year get a 15% discount. Workers who have served at least three years get

an additional 10% off the discounted price. How much does a worker who has served at least three years have to pay for boots?

    a. $63.78

    b. $64.65

    c. $71.83

    d. $72.05

Answer questions 51–53 on the basis of the following information.

This is to remind all sanitation workers that the two-way radios in the sanitation trucks are to be used for two purposes only—notification of irregular garbage pick-ups and report of emergencies. An irregular garbage pick-up is one where a worker comes upon an item that the worker is prohibited from picking up—for example, hazardous waste or a discarded appliance. Examples of an emergency are a truck breaking down or a worker's being sick or injured. Please remember that all other uses of the two-way radio are prohibited.

51. Sanitation Worker Burns is running behind schedule and is going to be late in picking up his daughter from school. According to the passage, he should NOT

    a. stop at a pay phone and call his daughter's school

    b. use the two-way radio to ask the dispatcher to call his daughter's school

    c. skip a few of his garbage pick-ups and get back on schedule

    d. let his daughter wait until he can get there

52. Sanitation truck number 97 is involved in an accident and, as a result, has a flat tire. The crew of the truck should

    a. ask the investigating police officer to notify the sanitation department

b. telephone the city maintenance department to send someone to change the tire

c. walk to a pay phone and call the shift supervisor

d. use the two-way radio to inform the dispatcher that the truck is broken down

53. The passage implies that

a. two-way radios have only recently been installed in the trucks

b. only some sanitation trucks have two-way radios

c. it is unusual for sanitation trucks to have two-way radios

d. some sanitation workers have been using the two-way radio improperly

Answer questions 54–56 solely on the basis of the following map. The arrows indicate traffic flow; one arrow indicates a one-way street going in the direction of the arrow; two arrows represent a two-way street. You are not allowed to go the wrong way on a one-way street.

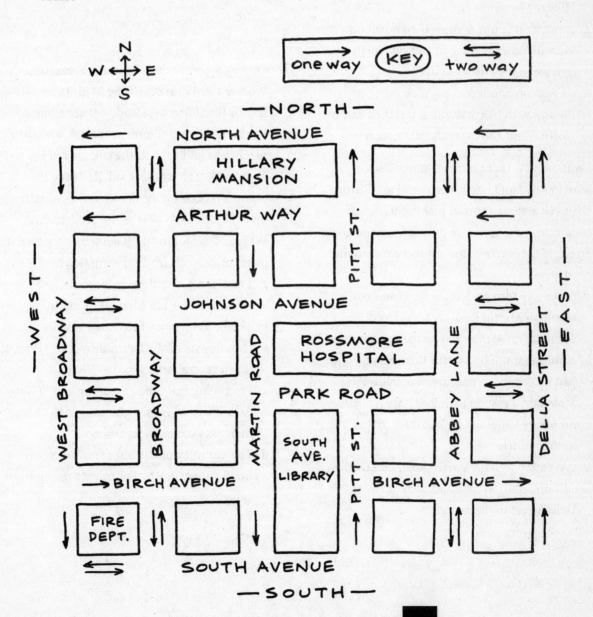

54. Sanitation Worker Lazar is spending his lunch break at the South Avenue Library, which faces South Avenue. His next garbage pick-up is at the Hillary Mansion, the entrance to which faces North Avenue. What is Lazar's most direct legal route to the Hillary Mansion?

a. go east on South Avenue, then north on Abbey Lane to North Avenue, and then west on North Avenue to the Hillary Mansion

b. go east on South Avenue, then north on Pitt Street, and then west on North Avenue to the Hillary Mansion

c. go west on South Avenue, then north on West Broadway, and then east on North Avenue to the Hillary Mansion

d. go west on South Avenue, then north on Broadway to North Avenue, and then east on North Avenue to the Hillary Mansion

55. Sanitation Worker Lowe is southbound on Martin Road and has just crossed Park Road. Dispatch assigns a special pick-up to him at a residence at the corner of Arthur Way and Della Street. What is Lowe's most direct route to the residence?

a. make a U-turn on Martin Road and go north on Martin Road to Arthur Way and then east on Arthur Way to the residence

b. continue south on Martin Road and then go east on South Avenue, then north on Pitt Street, then east on Park Road, then north on Abbey Lane, and then east on Arthur Way to the residence

c. continue south on Martin Road and then go east on South Avenue and then north on Della Street to the residence

d. continue south on Martin Road and then go east on Birch Avenue and then north on Della Street to the residence

56. Sanitation Worker Barker is heading west on Johnson Avenue. She makes a right turn on Broadway, a left turn on Arthur Way, a left turn onto West Broadway, and finally a left turn onto Birch Avenue. Which direction is Sanitation Worker Barker facing?

a. east

b. south

c. west

d. north

57. During a violent thunderstorm, Sanitation Worker Hernandez is sitting in his truck waiting for the storm to subside. He see a bolt of lightning, hears a thunderous crash, and then sees bricks falling from the chimney of the house at 770 Newfield Road. Realizing the house has been hit, he drives to the gas station up the block and calls the fire department. Which of the following statements reports the incident most clearly and accurately?

a. I'm at the gas station on Newfield Road where a house has been hit by lightning.

b. The house on Newfield Road just had its chimney struck by lightning, which knocked down several bricks.

c. I'm calling from the gas station at 770 Newfield Road, where the chimney of the house there was struck by lightning.

d. The chimney of the house at 770 Newfield Road was struck by lightning a few minutes ago.

58. Sanitation Worker Schultz is lifting a heavy garbage can at 9800 Commonwealth Boulevard when he feels a sharp pain in his back. He sets the can back down and then realizes that he can no longer stand up straight. He hobbles to the truck and calls the dispatcher. Which of the following reports most clearly and accurately describes what occurred?
a. My back was injured by the garbage can on Commonwealth Boulevard.
b. While I was lifting a can at 9800 Commonwealth Boulevard, I injured my back. I'm in pain and cannot stand up straight.
c. My back hurts and I cannot stand up when I was lifting a heavy can at 9800 Commonwealth Boulevard.
d. I felt a sharp pain in my back, which occurred at 9800 Commonwealth Boulevard, and I am calling to report that I am no longer standing.

59. You and your partner are loading a garbage barge. The load shifts suddenly and part of the garbage spills into the water. Your partner did not see what happened. What should you do?
a. load the rest of the garbage more carefully
b. stop loading and clean up the spill
c. clean up the spill only if someone complains
d. let the harbor police deal with the spill

60. While collecting trash in a residential neighborhood you see a man in dark clothing push in a side window and crawl into the house at 591 Oleander St. You believe no one is home because you saw two people drive away just a few minutes ago. What should you do?
a. keep working, because the situation might not be what it looks like
b. approach the window and ask the man who he is and what he is doing
c. sit in the truck and wait to see if the man comes out carrying stolen goods
d. use your truck radio to tell the dispatcher to call police to investigate

Answer questions 61 and 62 by choosing the word or phrase that means the same or nearly the same as the underlined word.

61. The residents of that area were <u>compliant</u> with the new rule about the proper disposal of broken glass.
a. skeptical
b. obedient
c. forgetful
d. appreciative

62. The general public seemed <u>apathetic</u> about the problem of improper waste disposal.
a. enraged
b. indifferent
c. suspicious
d. saddened

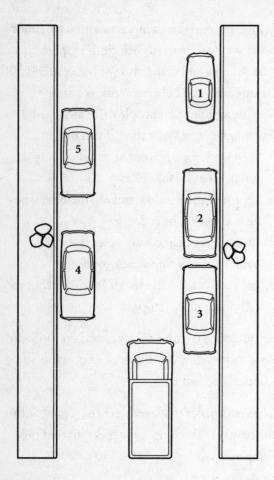

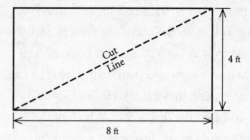

64. A four-foot by eight-foot sheet of plywood is cut into two pieces as shown above. What are the shapes of the two resulting pieces?
a. triangles
b. rectangles
c. squares
d. octagons

65. City regulations clearly state that sanitation workers do not have to pick up a can or bag that weighs more than 50 pounds. When Sanitation Worker Miller is making a pick-up on Linden Street, he attempts to pick up a can that is clearly overweight. He leaves a note for the resident. Which of the following most clearly and accurately describes the city's policy?
a. The city will not pick up any container that weighs more than 50 pounds.
b. This can weighs too much for me to pick up, which is part of the city's regulations of more than 50 pounds.
c. I will not pick up any can that weighs 50 pounds as this one.
d. On Linden Street, you have a can that weighs more than 50 pounds. I tried to pick it up, but I cannot due to city regulations.

63. On a one-way street such as that shown above, a collection truck may have to block the street briefly while garbage is collected. However, the truck driver should position the truck so that the handlers can pick up garbage quickly, yet without touching any cars parked on the street. In the scene shown above, where should the driver position the truck so that handlers can pick up both piles of garbage?
a. behind cars 2 and 3
b. parallel to car 4
c. parallel to car 1
d. in front of cars 1 and 5

Answer question 66 by choosing the word or phrase that means the same or nearly the same as the underlined word.

66. One of the duties of a shift supervisor is to <u>delegate</u> responsibility.
   a. analyze
   b. respect
   c. criticize
   d. assign

67. You are picking up garbage in a residential neighborhood when a man walks up to you and tells you he thinks sanitation workers have no right to be in unions because if they did their jobs right they wouldn't need to organize in order to be treated fairly. He then adds a bag to his pile of trash and goes back into his house. You are a union supporter. What should you do?
   a. refuse to pick up the trash the man put out, in order to teach him a lesson
   b. ring the man's bell and explain politely to him why unions are necessary
   c. call your supervisor and ask to have another worker assigned to this street
   d. ignore his comments and pick up his trash as you would anyone else's

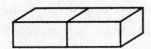

68. Which of the following figures (next column) could be the object above, seen from a different angle?

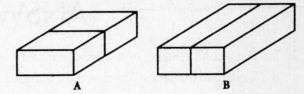
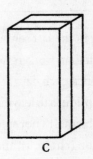

   a. C only
   b. A and B
   c. B and C
   d. A only

69. There are 176 men and 24 women employed as sanitation workers in District 4. What percentage of the district's sanitation workers is women?
   a. 12%
   b. 14%
   c. 16%
   d. 24%

70. Out of 100 city residents polled, 80 said they recycled their newspapers. How many residents out of 30,000 could be expected to recycle their newspapers?
   a. 2,400
   b. 6,000
   c. 20,000
   d. 24,000

ANSWER KEY

1. b. The second sentence of the passage indicates that sanitation workers will be cleaning the trucks.

2. d. The third sentence of the passage indicates that routes vary in the length of time they take to complete.

3. c. According to the last sentence of the passage, in the past sanitation workers usually were assigned to the same truck each day.

4. c. The best option is to let your supervisor know about the problem. It's not safe to drive the truck in this condition (choice a), and you would not be authorized to take it to an outside mechanic (choice b). You should not try to fix such a problem yourself (choice d), as this is the responsibility of the sanitation department's maintenance section.

5. b. It would be unsafe to go to work (choices a and c), as you would risk spreading the flu to your coworkers. Having another person call for you (choice d) might give the impression that you are not really sick.

6. a. Choice b does not say that Schmidt was injured; choices c and d are unclear.

7. a. The point on the graph for 1990 is closest to $6\frac{1}{2}$.

8. b. In both 1991 and 1992, the amount of garbage collected per truck per shift was 7 tons.

9. c. To solve the problem you have to first convert the time, 1 hour and 45 minutes, to minutes (60 minutes + 45 minutes = 105 minutes). Then multiply this by 4 (420 minutes), and then convert the answer back to hours by dividing by 60 minutes to arrive at the final answer (7 hours). Or you can multiply $1\frac{3}{4}$ hours by 4 to arrive at the same answer.

10. a. To solve the problem, multiply 3.5 pounds by 7, the number of days in one week.

11. c. Sentences three and four of the passage imply that all workers will be trained in the next six months. The passage implies that once workers are trained on the trucks, operation will not be limited to supervisors. The passage does not address issues of safety or seniority.

12. a. Sentences three and four of the passage indicate that special training is required to operate the automated garbage collection trucks. The issues raised in b, c, and d are not addressed by the passage.

13. d. Sentences three and four of the passage outline how sanitation workers will be trained on the new trucks.

14. b. According to the procedure, Lightsey's responsibility is to call for assistance immediately.

15. b. Finding a phone gives Upton a way to report an emergency such as this one. Ignoring the woman, who may be injured, would be irresponsible. The other two choices would waste valuable time.

16. d. Jessup should call for assistance on the truck radio, as the water will quickly become ice and pose a hazard to vehicles and pedestrians. Choice a would waste time. This *is* an emergency, so choice b is incorrect; however, the situation is not urgent enough to warrant dialing 911 (choice d).

17. c. This is the quickest way around the Ford Hotel and then to Cleveland Avenue. Choice a is not correct because it requires the sanitation workers to go the wrong way on Jones, a one-way street. Choice b would require the workers to drive through the Ford Hotel. Choice **d** has too many turns to be the most direct.

18. b. This choice is correct because it is the quickest and most direct route. Choice **a** has too many turns and takes the sanitation workers the wrong way on Adams Avenue. Lincoln Street is a one-way street going north, so choice **c** is wrong. Choice **d** takes the workers several blocks out of their way and so is not the most direct.

19. c. A right turn onto Glade Road turns Sanitation Worker Tonka west. The left onto Taft Road turns him south; the right onto Pine Avenue turns him west, the right onto Cleveland Avenue turns him back north, and then right onto Wilshire Avenue turns him east.

20. c. Figure #3 shows the attachment of the tie rod to the crankshaft at the bottom of the crankshaft. Another 90-degree counterclockwise rotation would place the attachment point on the right side of the crankshaft at position C.

21. c. When an employee is *accountable* for something, he or she is *responsible* for it.

22. c. It's best not to interrupt your schedule or the flow of your work just to chat (choices **a** and **b**), and your friend will probably understand if you keep the conversation brief. Asking someone else to do your job so you can stop to talk (choice **d**) would never be a good option.

23. a. It's best to get a different spreader through the proper channels. The other options could be dangerous, as hazard lights are an important safety device.

24. b. Choices **a** and **d** leave out important information; choice **c** is inaccurate.

25. c. Choice **a** is inaccurate because it indicates that the car is three weeks old. Choice **b** gives an incorrect license number. Choice **d** leaves out important information.

26. a. The rule states th... see if anyone involved... call for a supervisor.

27. d. Since an injury has o... for medical help first and... supervisor.

28. b. Two weeks after June 8 is...

29. a. *Diplomatic* means *tactful.*

30. b. You should not take respons... yourself (options **a** and **c**), as th... equipped to handle the problem. L... with a stranger (choice **d**) could be...

31. c. The barrel is round and should r... other items would have to be pick... carried.

32. b. Driving in winter weather requires... take things slowly, so choice **a** is incorrect. T... means that you should be cautious because o... sible icy conditions, but it does not prohibit... from driving on the bridge, so choice **c** would... inappropriate. Pumping the brakes (choice **d**)... not a safe option, as it could actually cause a skid...

33. d. Choices **a** and **b** do not explain the fee accurately. The second sentence in choice **c** is unclear.

34. a. Choices **b** and **c** leave out information; choice **d** is unclear.

35. d. The area is the length times the width ($A = LW$). So you must multiply: 42 times 40 is 1680.

36. a. First it is necessary to convert centimeters to inches. To do this for choice **a**, multiply 100 cm by 0.39 inches, yielding 39 inches. For choice **b**, 1 yard is 36 inches. For choice **d**, multiply 85 cm by 0.39 inches, yielding 33.15 inches. Choice **a**, 1 meter (or 39 inches), is the longest.

37. d. Sweeping around the car is the best you can do under these circumstances. Trying to find the owner (choice **a**) would waste time unnecessarily. Choice **b** would be illegal and unsafe. There is no

c. Divide 135 Spanish-speaking employees by
125 total employees to arrive at 0.12, or 12%.

can't just take 25% off the original price,
the 10% discount after three years of ser-
s taken off the price that has already been
duced by 15%. Figure the problem in two steps:
after the 15% discount, the price is $71.83. Ninety
percent of that—subtracting 10%—is $64.65.

51. b. Although choices c and d may be inappropriate responses to the situation, the passage only
specifically prohibits choice b, using the two-way
radio.

52. d. One of the two appropriate uses of the two-way
radio mentioned in the passage is *report of emergencies.*

53. d. The first sentence of the passage says its purpose
is to remind sanitation workers of the proper use
of the radios. This implies that some workers have
been using the radio improperly. The passage does
not allude to how recently the radios have been
installed (choice a), how many trucks have them
(choice b), or how common they are (choice c).

54. a. This the most direct route to the Hillary Mansion, requiring the fewest changes in direction.
Choice b requires Sanitation Worker Lazar to
drive through the Rossmore Hospital. Choice c
takes him the wrong way on West Broadway and
North Avenue. Choice d takes Lazar the wrong way
on North Avenue.

55. c. This route requires the fewest number of turns.
Choice a is wrong because Martin Road is a one-
way street. Choice b requires a number of turns
and goes the wrong way on Arthur Way. Choice d
would require Sanitation Worker Lowe to drive
through the South Avenue Library.

56. a. A right turn onto Broadway turns Sanitation
Worker Barker north. The left turn onto Arthur
Way turns her back west, the left turn onto West

at Gonzales should check to
needs medical help and then
curred, Kare should call
then call a department
June 22.
bility for the child
e police are best
eaving the child
dangerous.
ll easily; the
ed up and
that you
he sign
f pos-
you
be
is

workers to
en a truck is

up without another
partner is there to help.
nnecessary waste of time.
ght be dangerous

problem, divide the number of
by the number of kilograms in a
2): 168 divided by 2.2 is 76.3. Now
o the nearest unit, which is 76.

60% of the residents were fined, 40% were
ot fined. Forty percent of 220 is 88.

b. Choice a is inaccurate; choice c is unclear;
choice d leaves out information.

46. d. The only sensible option is to call police immediately. Nothing should be disturbed, because this
is a crime scene.

47. a. Although it is unpleasant to get someone you
work with in trouble, a coworker who is intoxicated
poses a threat to your safety and to his. This is a
problem for a supervisor to handle.

48. c. Choice a distorts what really happened. Choice
b gives inaccurate information. Choice d implies
that the woman in the Toyota was driving the
wrong way.

Broadway turns her south, and the left turn onto Birch Avenue turns her east.

57. **d.** Choices **a** and **c** are inaccurate; choice **b** leaves out the complete address.

58. **b.** Choice **a** is unclear and incomplete. Choice **c** is unclear, and choice **d** is inaccurate and incomplete.

59. **b.** Part of being a good employee is taking responsibility for one's job, and you would not be doing this if you ignored the problem (as choices **a** and **c** imply). Letting someone else handle this problem (choice **d**) would be unprofessional.

60. **d.** As a responsible member of society, you should call the police. The man's dark clothing and his entering a side window are suspicious, so ignoring the situation or waiting to see if he comes out carrying stolen goods (choices **a** and **c**) are not sensible options. Approaching the window and confronting the man (choice **b**) could be very dangerous.

61. **b.** When people are *compliant* with a rule, they are *obedient*.

62. **b.** *Apathetic* means *indifferent*.

63. **c.** Parking parallel to car 1 will enable the handlers to carry the pile of garbage on the left side of the street through the gap between cars 4 and 5 and the pile of garbage on the right side through the gap between cars 1 and 2.

64. **a.** The resulting shapes are three-sided closed polygons, or triangles.

65. **a.** Choice **b** is unclear; choice **c** does not indicate that this is a city regulation; choice **d** is unclear.

66. **d.** To *delegate* responsibility is to *assign* it to someone else.

67. **d.** Ignoring the man's comments and continuing with your duties is the most professional option. To overreact (choices **a** and **c**) would be unprofessional. To follow the man and engage him in further debate (choice **b**) would take you away from your work and waste time.

68. **d.** Figure A is the object shown as seen from the end.

69. **a.** Add the number of men and women to get the total number of sanitation workers: 200. The number of women, 24, is 12% of 200.

70. **d.** Eighty out of 100 is 80%. Eighty percent of 30,000 is 24,000.

SCORING

In order to score your exam, begin by counting the total number of questions you got right out of the 70 questions on the test. Next, you have to convert that score into a percentage. Divide your correct answer score by 0.7 to get the total percentage of right answers. The table below will help you check your math by giving you percentage equivalents for several possible scores.

Number of questions right	Approximate percentage
70	100%
65	93%
60	86%
55	79%
50	71%
45	64%
40	57%
35	50%

You need a score of at least 70 percent to pass the Sanitation Worker exam in most cities. You have probably seen improvement between your first practice exam score and this one. Here's what you should do next, based on your score on this exam:

- **If you scored below 50 percent,** you should do some serious thinking about whether you're really ready to take the Sanitation Worker exam. An adult education course in reading comprehension at a high school or community college would be a very good strategy. If you don't have time for a course, you should at least try to get some private tutoring.
- **If your score is in the 50 to 70 percent range,** you need to work as hard as you can in the time you

have left to boost your skills. Consider the LearningExpress book *Reading Comprehension in 20 Minutes a Day* (order information at the back of this book) or other books from your public library. Also, re-read Chapters 6–10 of this book, and make sure you take *all* of the advice there for improving your score. Enlist friends and family to help you by making up mock test questions and quizzing you on them.

- **If your score is between 70 and 80 percent,** you could still benefit from additional work to just to make sure you score above 70 percent on the real test. Go back to Chapters 6–10 and study them carefully.
- **If you scored above 80 percent,** congratulations! You may want to review this book a bit before the exam, just for insurance, but basically, you should start concentrating on making sure you're ready for the physical test.

If you didn't score as well as you would like, try to analyze the reasons why. Did you run out of time before you could answer all the questions? Did you go back and change your answer from the right one to a wrong one? Did you get flustered and sit staring at a hard question for what seemed like hours? If you had any of these problems, go back and review the test-taking strategies in Chapter 4 to learn how to avoid them.

You should also look at how you did on each kind of question on the test if you still need to improve your score. You may have done very well on reading comprehension questions and poorly on math questions, or vice versa. If you can figure out where your strengths and weaknesses lie, you'll know where to concentrate your efforts in the time you have left before the exam. The table on the next page identifies which questions on the practice exam fall into which categories and tells you which chapters to review if you had trouble with a particular type.

Once you've done as much as you can to get ready for the exam, take the third practice exam in Chapter 12. Treat it as if it were the real exam, and then you'll really know how well prepared you are.

Question type	Question numbers	Chapter
Understanding written language	1–3, 7, 8, 11–13, 28, 39–41, 51–53	6, "Reading Comprehension"
Communicating information	6, 21, 24, 25, 29, 33, 34, 45, 48, 57, 58, 61, 62, 65, 66	7, "Verbal Expression"
Using spatial reasoning	17–20, 31, 54–56, 63, 64, 68	8, "Map Reading and Spatial Relations"
Using judgment and following rules	4, 5, 14–16, 22, 23, 26, 27, 30, 32, 37, 38, 42, 46, 47, 59, 60, 67	9, "Good Judgment and Common Sense"
Math	9, 10, 35, 36, 43, 44, 49, 50, 69, 70	10, "Math"

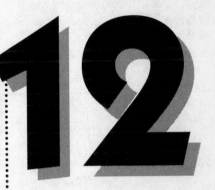

C·H·A·P·T·E·R

SANITATION WORKER PRACTICE EXAM 3

12

CHAPTER SUMMARY

This is the third of three practice exams in this book based on the most commonly tested areas on sanitation worker written exams across the country. By now, you have worked through the instructional material in the previous chapters and have taken the second practice exam. Use this third exam to see how much your score has improved since you took the second one.

A s noted, the actual exam you take may be somewhat different from the ones in this book; however, you should find that most of the same skills are tested on the real exam as on these practice exams. This test, like the previous two, includes 70 multiple-choice questions on reading comprehension, verbal expression, mathematics, judgment and application of procedure, spatial relations, and map-reading.

Once again, try to come as close to the actual test-taking experience as you possibly can. Work in a quiet place where you won't be interrupted. Tear out the answer sheet on the next page and fill in the circles with your number 2 pencils. Give yourself two hours for the entire exam, using a timer or stopwatch.

After the exam, again use the answer key that follows it to see how you did. The answer explanations in that section should be helpful for any question you missed. After the answer key is a section on scoring your exam.

1.	ⓐ	ⓑ	ⓒ	ⓓ	26.	ⓐ	ⓑ	ⓒ	ⓓ	51.	ⓐ	ⓑ	ⓒ	ⓓ
2.	ⓐ	ⓑ	ⓒ	ⓓ	27.	ⓐ	ⓑ	ⓒ	ⓓ	52.	ⓐ	ⓑ	ⓒ	ⓓ
3.	ⓐ	ⓑ	ⓒ	ⓓ	28.	ⓐ	ⓑ	ⓒ	ⓓ	53.	ⓐ	ⓑ	ⓒ	ⓓ
4.	ⓐ	ⓑ	ⓒ	ⓓ	29.	ⓐ	ⓑ	ⓒ	ⓓ	54.	ⓐ	ⓑ	ⓒ	ⓓ
5.	ⓐ	ⓑ	ⓒ	ⓓ	30.	ⓐ	ⓑ	ⓒ	ⓓ	55.	ⓐ	ⓑ	ⓒ	ⓓ
6.	ⓐ	ⓑ	ⓒ	ⓓ	31.	ⓐ	ⓑ	ⓒ	ⓓ	56.	ⓐ	ⓑ	ⓒ	ⓓ
7.	ⓐ	ⓑ	ⓒ	ⓓ	32.	ⓐ	ⓑ	ⓒ	ⓓ	57.	ⓐ	ⓑ	ⓒ	ⓓ
8.	ⓐ	ⓑ	ⓒ	ⓓ	33.	ⓐ	ⓑ	ⓒ	ⓓ	58.	ⓐ	ⓑ	ⓒ	ⓓ
9.	ⓐ	ⓑ	ⓒ	ⓓ	34.	ⓐ	ⓑ	ⓒ	ⓓ	59.	ⓐ	ⓑ	ⓒ	ⓓ
10.	ⓐ	ⓑ	ⓒ	ⓓ	35.	ⓐ	ⓑ	ⓒ	ⓓ	60.	ⓐ	ⓑ	ⓒ	ⓓ
11.	ⓐ	ⓑ	ⓒ	ⓓ	36.	ⓐ	ⓑ	ⓒ	ⓓ	61.	ⓐ	ⓑ	ⓒ	ⓓ
12.	ⓐ	ⓑ	ⓒ	ⓓ	37.	ⓐ	ⓑ	ⓒ	ⓓ	62.	ⓐ	ⓑ	ⓒ	ⓓ
13.	ⓐ	ⓑ	ⓒ	ⓓ	38.	ⓐ	ⓑ	ⓒ	ⓓ	63.	ⓐ	ⓑ	ⓒ	ⓓ
14.	ⓐ	ⓑ	ⓒ	ⓓ	39.	ⓐ	ⓑ	ⓒ	ⓓ	64.	ⓐ	ⓑ	ⓒ	ⓓ
15.	ⓐ	ⓑ	ⓒ	ⓓ	40.	ⓐ	ⓑ	ⓒ	ⓓ	65.	ⓐ	ⓑ	ⓒ	ⓓ
16.	ⓐ	ⓑ	ⓒ	ⓓ	41.	ⓐ	ⓑ	ⓒ	ⓓ	66.	ⓐ	ⓑ	ⓒ	ⓓ
17.	ⓐ	ⓑ	ⓒ	ⓓ	42.	ⓐ	ⓑ	ⓒ	ⓓ	67.	ⓐ	ⓑ	ⓒ	ⓓ
18.	ⓐ	ⓑ	ⓒ	ⓓ	43.	ⓐ	ⓑ	ⓒ	ⓓ	68.	ⓐ	ⓑ	ⓒ	ⓓ
19.	ⓐ	ⓑ	ⓒ	ⓓ	44.	ⓐ	ⓑ	ⓒ	ⓓ	69.	ⓐ	ⓑ	ⓒ	ⓓ
20.	ⓐ	ⓑ	ⓒ	ⓓ	45.	ⓐ	ⓑ	ⓒ	ⓓ	70.	ⓐ	ⓑ	ⓒ	ⓓ
21.	ⓐ	ⓑ	ⓒ	ⓓ	46.	ⓐ	ⓑ	ⓒ	ⓓ					
22.	ⓐ	ⓑ	ⓒ	ⓓ	47.	ⓐ	ⓑ	ⓒ	ⓓ					
23.	ⓐ	ⓑ	ⓒ	ⓓ	48.	ⓐ	ⓑ	ⓒ	ⓓ					
24.	ⓐ	ⓑ	ⓒ	ⓓ	49.	ⓐ	ⓑ	ⓒ	ⓓ					
25.	ⓐ	ⓑ	ⓒ	ⓓ	50.	ⓐ	ⓑ	ⓒ	ⓓ					

SANITATION WORKER EXAM 3

Answer questions 1 and 2 based on the rule below.

It's important to know the height of your truck before you start your route. The truck you are driving may be too tall to fit underneath an overhead object such as a power line. If you aren't sure that you will fit under an overhead object, you must stop, get out of the truck, and look. If you see that the object is hanging too low, find a way around the obstacle.

1. Early one morning Sanitation Worker Wallace is traveling down Palm Drive, a four-lane roadway. He notices that the heavy storm last night has caused power lines to sag, and there are tree limbs scattered in the street. At one intersection he sees that the overhead signal light has sagged dangerously low. What should he do?
   a. slow down enough so that, if the truck bumps it, the light will slide harmlessly along the top of the truck
   b. pull over and wait until a truck as tall as his tries to go through the intersection first
   c. signal and move carefully into a lane that will allow him to miss hitting the signal light
   d. get out and measure the distance from the ground to the light with a tape measure

2. Sanitation Worker Ammand's truck has broken down, and he is using the new spare truck to finish out his route. He is coming up on an intersection where the overhang of an old building extends out into the narrow street, and he's not sure the truck will fit under it. What should he do?

   a. stop and get out of the truck to assess whether it will fit under the overhang before making the turn
   b. watch for pedestrians and then ease the truck onto the sidewalk to get around the overhang
   c. back the truck up and skip picking up garbage on this street until his regular truck is available
   d. ask the dispatcher to call the building owner to find out the height of the overhang

3. On his way to work at 6:40 a.m., Sanitation Worker Marshall's car gets a flat tire. He manages to pull the car over to the shoulder of the road and decides he will change the tire himself. Though his shift begins at 7:00 a.m., he now estimates that he will not arrive on the job until about 7:20 a.m. He phones his supervisor from a public telephone to report that he will be late. Which of the following reports most clearly and accurately describes the situation?
   a. I was driving to work. I won't be there until about 20 minutes later than was expected.
   b. On my way to work, there was a flat tire, which I am about to fix. It is now about 6:40.
   c. I would have been on time, but now I am unable to make it by 7:00 because the car is on the shoulder of the road.
   d. I am stuck on the side of the road with a flat tire. I will change it and should be in around 7:20.

4. Highway Route Markers: Even numbers indicate east-west interstate routes while odd numbers indicate north-south routes. Interstate highways identified by a three-digit number are usually alternate or bypass routes. Which of the following is an east-west route?
   a. Interstate 5
   b. Interstate 29
   c. Interstate 35
   d. Interstate 80

5. Your truck is full and you've just made your last pickup. The final load contained a large wooden crate that sticks out of the top of your truck by two feet. As you drive down a residential street you see that a high-voltage power line, coated with ice, is sagging a bit lower than usual. What should you do?
   a. get out of the truck and look to make sure that the crate will fit under the power line
   b. keep driving very slowly so that if the crate hits the power line the line will bounce off
   c. have your helper stand on top of the crate and move the power line up as you drive carefully underneath it
   d. call the power company and wait for them to come tighten up the line before you proceed

6. Department regulations require collection trucks to have transmission maintenance every 13,000 miles. Truck #B-17 last had maintenance on its transmission at 12,398 miles. The mileage gauge now reads 22,003. How many more miles can the truck be driven before it must be brought in for transmission maintenance?

   a. 3,395
   b. 4,395
   c. 9,003
   d. 9,605

Answer question 7 based on the passage below.

Every year Americans use over one billion sharp objects to administer health care in their homes. These sharp objects include lancets, needles, and syringes. If not disposed of in puncture-resistant containers, they can injure sanitation workers. Sharp objects should be disposed of in hard plastic or metal containers with secure lids. The containers should be clearly marked and be puncture resistant.

7. According to the passage, injuries can occur to sanitation workers if they
   a. pick up plastic or metal objects that have been placed in soft plastic bags
   b. come into contact with sharp objects not placed in secure containers
   c. use sharp objects such as lancets, needles, and syringes in their homes
   d. have not marked containers that have been filled with sharp objects

8. An employee handbook states, "If you are sick and unable to report to work on any given day, you must notify your supervisor at least one hour prior to the start of your shift." If your shift begins each day at 7:30 a.m., this means that

a. if you cannot be at work, you must notify your supervisor by 6:30 a.m. that same day

b. if you get sick during working hours, you must notify your supervisor an hour before you want to leave for home

c. all workers who are sick and have not notified their supervisors by 7:30 must report to work no later than 8:30

d. when you are sick you must phone your supervisor by 8:30 a.m. each morning

9. You have been assigned to a new route. After your first pickup, you see that you have to back up your truck 10 feet to get out of a narrow alley. The mirror mounted on the passenger side of the truck has been bumped out of position so that you can't see behind the truck. What should you do?

a. keep backing up—you can use the mirror on the driver's side of the truck to back safely

b. stop, open the door on your side so you can see out, and then back up, honking about every three feet

c. keep looking straight ahead at the front of the truck so that you can tell if the wheels are rolling straight while backing

d. stop, adjust the mirror so that you can see behind the truck, and then continue backing slowly

10. Sanitation Worker Rivers is approaching the intersection at First Street and Wayne Avenue when he notices that the stoplight is not operating. Because this is a busy intersection and a potentially dangerous situation, Rivers stops at the nearest public telephone and calls the police department. Which of the following reports most clearly and accurately describes the situation?

a. As I was driving along First Street toward Wayne, I noticed a dangerous situation and decided to report it.

b. The light would not turn red at the intersection of First Street.

c. The stoplight is not working at the intersection of First Street and Wayne Avenue.

d. Traffic is a problem on Wayne Avenue, where the stoplight may have been broken.

11. They heard <u>intermittent</u> rattling of trash receptacles all night long, thought to be caused by foraging raccoons. In this sentence, the word <u>intermittent</u> most nearly means

a. protracted

b. periodic

c. disquieting

d. vehement

Answer questions 12 and 13 based on the procedure below.

Lifting trash can easily strain the backs of sanitation workers. Before lifting, workers are asked to get a feel for how heavy the trash is by tipping the container back and forth or pulling lightly at the bag. To keep from straining back muscles, workers should keep both feet flat on the ground while lifting. To avoid back injuries, workers are also asked *not* to lock their knees when lifting. If a container is too heavy, a worker should not attempt to lift it without the help of another worker.

12. Sanitation Worker Spagenberg has drawn the truck up close to a container of trash and has gotten out. He now stands with one foot in the gutter and one foot on the sidewalk. The container is large and looks quite heavy. What should he do next?

a. brace himself firmly and pull the container up into his arms

b. step onto the sidewalk and tip the container a bit to see how heavy it is

c. pull the container over into the gutter and then lift it into the truck

d. skip this apparently heavy container and come back with help

13. Sanitation Worker Graviel must lift a large, rather heavy cardboard box onto the truck. How should she pick up the box?

a. lock both knees and bend over at the waist

b. bend over at the waist and drag it

c. sit down on the curb, pull the box into her lap, and then stand upright

d. face the box, keep both feet flat on the ground, and bend her knees

Answer questions 14 through 16 based on the chart below.

Correct Disposal Method for Hazardous Waste Materials

- ♣   Dry out and put in trash
- ●   Pour down sewer system
- ♦   Hazardous: save for special collection

Ant poison		♦
Aerosol cans	♣	
Bathroom cleaner		●
Bug spray		♦
Furniture polish	♣	
Medicine (expired)		♦
Nail polish	♣	
Oven cleaner		♦
Skin cream	♣	
Window cleaner		●
Antifreeze		●
Battery acid		♦
Brake fluid		♦
Fuel oil		♦
Gasoline		♦
Paint—latex	♣	
Paint—oil based	♣	
Varnish		♦

14. According to the chart, which of the following should be dried out and placed in the trash?

a. window cleaner

b. antifreeze

c. oil-based paint

d. expired medicine

15. What is the correct method for disposing of an aerosol can that is half full of bug spray?
   a. place it in the trash
   b. save it until there is a special collection
   c. empty the spray into the sewer system
   d. spray it onto a hard surface and let it evaporate into the air

16. Which of the following may be correctly disposed of by pouring it into the sewer system?
   a. bathroom cleaner
   b. furniture polish
   c. gasoline
   d. latex paint

17. A truck carrying a load of debris weighs $5\frac{1}{2}$ tons. The same truck, when empty, weighs 3 tons. What is the weight of the load?
   a. $2\frac{1}{2}$ tons
   b. 3 tons
   c. $3\frac{1}{4}$ tons
   d. $3\frac{1}{2}$ tons

18. Sanitation Worker Jarvis is heading east across the Livingston Bridge. There had been rain earlier in the day, but now the temperature has dropped below freezing. Halfway across the bridge, his truck hits a patch of ice and slides into a guard rail. Fortunately, Jarvis is not hurt. There is slight damage, however, to the right side of the truck. Later, Jarvis files a report on the accident. Which of the following reports describes the incident most clearly and accurately?
   a. The guard rail damaged the right side of the truck, which was sitting on the Livingston Bridge on a patch of ice.
   b. As I was driving on the Livingston Bridge, I hit some ice and slid into a guard rail, damaging the right side of the truck.
   c. When I hit an icy patch along the Livingston Bridge, the guard rail hit the right side of the truck, causing me to slide into it.
   d. Though I was not hurt, the truck was on its side after it hit the guard rail on the bridge.

19. You have been assigned to a truck as a helper. Your main responsibility is to direct the driver when she's backing up the truck. On your first stop it begins to rain hard, but the driver needs to back up about six feet after picking up a load. What should you do?
   a. stay inside the truck and help by watching the right mirror
   b. sit and wait until the rain stops
   c. ask the driver to get out and check behind the vehicle
   d. get out of the truck and guide her back safely

20. You and your helper are at either end of an old sofa, carrying it to the truck. As both of you start to lift the sofa into the rear of the truck, your helper tells you his back hurts and he doesn't think he can hold onto the sofa. What should you do?
   a. set the sofa down immediately and get medical attention for your helper
   b. tell the helper to keep lifting, but to drop it if he finds he absolutely can't do it
   c. both of you take the sofa back to the curb and leave it for another crew
   d. ask a nearby pedestrian to help put the sofa in the truck

Answer questions 21 and 22 based on the passage and the calendar below.

JUNE						
S	**M**	**T**	**W**	**Th**	**F**	**S**
1	2	3	4	5	6	7
8	9	10	11	12	13	14
15	16	17	18	19	20	21
22	23	24	25	26	27	28
29	30					

An employee who has just been hired receives a notice that states, "All new employees must have a medical examination before they begin work. Medical exams are given at the health clinic at 1641 Adams Street on the first and third Tuesdays and the first and third Fridays of each month, beginning at 11:00 a.m."

21. According to the notice, an employee who is hired on June 4 and plans to begin work on June 16 must have a medical exam on
   a. June 6
   b. June 10
   c. June 13
   d. June 17

22. According to the notice, which of the following is a day when medical exams are NOT given?
   a. June 3
   b. June 17
   c. June 20
   d. June 24

23. Drivers must report the mileage on their trucks each week. The mileage reading of vehicle #A-23 was 20,907 at the beginning of one week, and 21,053 at the end of the same week. What was the total number of miles driven that week?
   a. 46
   b. 145
   c. 146
   d. 156

24. Sanitation Worker Caruso is loading a collection truck with trash in front of the apartment building at 3232 Atlantic Street when nine-year-old Joey Tremont asks if he would help pull a kitten down from a nearby tree. Caruso sees that he can easily reach the limb where the kitten is trapped. As he is pulling the kitten to safety, the kitten scratches him on the face. The next day, Caruso's face is swollen, and the scratch has become infected. He must file a medical report. Which of the following reports describes the incident most clearly and accurately?
   a. A kitten scratched me as I was making a pickup in front of the apartment building at 3232 Atlantic Street. The boy's name was Joey.
   b. Joey Tremont asked me to save his kitten, but when I did, he scratched me in the face and became infected.

c. While I was collecting at 3232 Atlantic Street, a boy named Joey asked me to rescue his kitten from a tree. As I was lifting the kitten, it scratched me, and the scratch is now infected.

d. Having rescued a kitten from a tree, which was owned by a boy named Joey, I was scratched in the face. This took place at a collection stop at the apartment building on Atlantic Street. Then it became infected.

Answer questions 25 and 26 based on the passage below.

You should be aware of your limitations as a driver. You are responsible for what your vehicle does. Fatigue, stress, and illness will affect your driving. Being tired is a bigger problem at night. Drivers who are not alert may not react as quickly to hazards. If you are sleepy, the only safe cure is to get off the road.

25. According to the passage, when drivers are fatigued, they
   a. become ill
   b. are not as alert
   c. have too much stress
   d. drive off the road

26. According to the passage, if, while driving, you feel as though you are falling asleep, you should
   a. drive more slowly
   b. drive more carefully
   c. drink coffee
   d. stop driving

27. Sanitation Workers Ellis and Wong are collecting trash in the alley behind the building at 1412 Longview Avenue when Wong notices a suspicious-looking receptacle in one of the dumpsters. When Ellis agrees that this receptacle may possibly contain an explosive, the two workers immediately follow department policy by leaving the area and phoning the police. Which of the following reports describes the situation most clearly and accurately?
   a. There may be an explosive in a dumpster in the alley behind 1412 Longview Avenue.
   b. Something looks suspicious at 1412 Longview Avenue, which could possibly explode.
   c. There is a receptacle in a dumpster in the alley on Longview Avenue, and it is in the trash we were about to collect.
   d. At 1412 Longview Avenue, there is something suspicious-looking sitting behind it in the dumpster in the alley.

Answer questions 28 and 29 based on the map below.

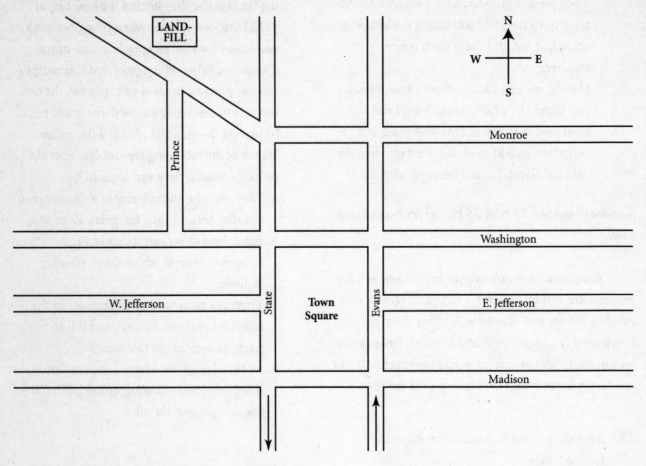

As indicated, State Street is one-way going south, and Evans Street is one-way going north. All other streets have two-way traffic.

28. A special collection truck is headed east on West Jefferson on its way to a pickup at the corner of Evans and East Jefferson. In order to travel the shortest distance without breaking traffic laws, the truck should turn
   a. right onto State, right onto Washington, right onto Evans
   b. left onto State, left onto Madison, left onto Evans

   c. right onto State, left onto Madison, left onto Evans
   d. left onto State, left onto Evans, right onto East Jefferson

29. A collection truck is headed in the direction of the landfill, which is located just off Monroe Street. The truck is already on Monroe, stopped at a red light at the intersection of Monroe and State. To reach the landfill, in which direction will the truck travel?
   a. northeast
   b. northwest
   c. southeast
   d. southwest

30. You are driving a garbage truck called a "front end loader." You pick up dumpsters with this truck by using equipment located on the front of your truck. A helper is along and usually only directs you when you have to back up the truck. Today, bright sunlight is creating such a glare on your front windshield that you cannot see the next dumpster as you and your helper pull up near it. What should you do?

    a. have the helper run around to the rear of the truck and check to see what is behind the truck

    b. have the helper walk to the front of the truck and direct you up to the dumpster

    c. hold one hand in front of your eyes to cut the glare and then pull on up to the dumpster

    d. drive forward very slowly and carefully, until you feel the truck bump the dumpster, then get out and look to see if you connected properly

31. City Worker Lopez was operating a street sweeper in the middle of the 2200 block of Howard Street when a woman suddenly ran up to the vehicle. The woman, Ina Barry, explained that she was certain her gold watch had fallen into the street the previous evening. Then she accused Lopez of having swept up the watch with the street sweeper. She wanted him to look for it immediately. Lopez told her to phone the Sanitation Department and file a report. That afternoon, Lopez also reported the incident. Which of the following describes the incident most clearly and accurately?

    a. Ina Barry is the name of the woman who said I had stolen a gold watch from her in the middle of 2200 Howard Street.

    b. While I was working at 220 Howard Street, I told a woman named Ina Barry to file a report with the Sanitation Department about her watch.

    c. The street sweeper I was operating in the 2200 block of Howard Street picked up Ina Barry's gold watch when I told her to file a report with the department.

    d. As I was sweeping the 2200 block of Howard Street, Ina Barry ran up and accused me of having swept up her gold watch.

32. If a vehicle is driven 21 miles on Monday, 18 miles on Tuesday, and 24 miles on Wednesday, what is the average number of miles driven each day?

    a. 19

    b. 21

    c. 22

    d. 23.5

Answer question 33 based on the passage below.

A job announcement states, "The application period for this position is from January 15 through March 1. Applications are available at the City Department of Sanitation. Application forms must be *received* at the department by 5:00 p.m. on the closing date of the application period."

33. Which of the following persons has NOT met the requirements of the job announcement?
  a. Ron picks up an application on February 22, completes it, and drops it in the mail just before 5:00 p.m. on March 1.
  b. Joan picks up an application on March 1, completes it, and returns it to the City Department of Sanitation at 4:30 p.m. the same day.
  c. Samuel completes an application and mails it to the Department of Sanitation on January 16.
  d. Alicia picks up an application, completes it, and returns it to the City Department of Sanitation at 2:00 p.m. on March 1.

34. The city gave <u>tentative</u> approval to the recycling plan. In this sentence, the word <u>tentative</u> most nearly means
  a. provisional
  b. ambiguous
  c. wholehearted
  d. unnecessary

Answer questions 35 and 36 based on the chart below.

LOADS OF TRASH DUMPED DURING THE WEEK OF AUGUST 3					
Truck	**M**	**T**	**W**	**Th**	**F**
B-209	5	6	5	7	4
G-648	3	6	5	5	5
K-121	7	5	5	8	4
M-459	4	5	5	6	6

35. On which day did all four trucks dump the same number of loads?
  a. Tuesday
  b. Wednesday
  c. Thursday
  d. Friday

36. The truck that dumped the greatest number of loads on Friday was
  a. B-209
  b. G-648
  c. K-121
  d. M-459

Answer question 37 based on the map below.

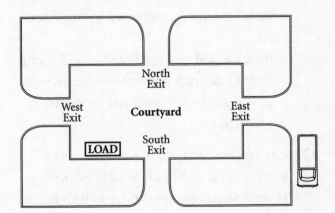

37. Which exit should a worker use to carry the load the shortest distance to the back of the truck?
  a. North
  b. South
  c. West
  d. East

38. When the Franklins told scientists that a UFO had landed behind their dumpster, the scientists were <u>incredulous</u>. In this sentence, the word <u>incredulous</u> most nearly means
 a. outraged
 b. stunned
 c. disbelieving
 d. delighted

Answer questions 39 through 44 based on Diagram D and the information below.

Diagram D is a map of a section of the city, where some public buildings are located. Each of the squares represent one city block. Street names are as shown. If there is an arrow next to the street name, it means the street is one way only in the direction of the arrow. If there is no arrow next to the street name, two-way traffic is allowed.

39. Sanitation Workers Rao and Morgan have just made a pickup between the clinic and the fire house when they are called to make a special pickup at the corner of Brown Street and 9th Avenue. What is the most direct legal way for them to travel?
 a. east on Maple Street and north on 9th Avenue to the pickup site
 b. west on Maple Street, north on 12th Avenue, and east on Brown Street to the pickup site
 c. east on Maple Street and north on 11th Avenue to the pickup site
 d. west on Maple Street, north on 11th Avenue, and east on Brown Street to the pickup site

40. What streets run north and south of the park?
 a. Brown Street and Oak Street
 b. Maple Street and Park Street

 c. Brown Street and Park Street
 d. Green Street and Oak Street

41. A person leaving the clinic needs to go to the drug store. If you were giving her driving directions from the clinic, what would be the most direct route?
 a. east on Maple Street, north on 9th Avenue, and west on Brown Street to the store entrance
 b. west on Maple Street, north on 10th Avenue, and west on Brown Street to the store entrance
 c. west on Green Street, north on 12th Avenue, and east on Brown Street to the store entrance
 d. east on Oak Street, north on 11th Avenue, and east on Brown Street to the store entrance

42. Someone has committed vandalism at the junior high school by strewing trash over the school grounds. You have been asked to make a special pickup at the school, then proceed to your regular pickup at the hospital. What is the best route for you to take from school to hospital?
 a. north on 10th Avenue, west on Brown Street, and south on 12th Avenue to the hospital entrance
 b. south on 10th Avenue and west on Green Street to the hospital entrance
 c. north on 10th Avenue and south on Brown Street to the hospital entrance
 d. south on 10th Avenue, south on Maple Street, and east on Green Street to the hospital entrance

Diagram D

Expressway

N
W — E
S

BROWN STREET

GAS STATION

DRUG STORE

PARK

OAK STREET

PARK

JUNIOR HIGH SCHOOL

STREET

12th AVENUE

11th AVENUE

10th AVENUE

9th AVENUE

LIBRARY

POLICE STATION

MAPLE STREET

HOSPITAL

FIRE HOUSE

CLINIC

GREEN STREET

43. You have just made a pickup from the dumpster at the fire house and need to fill your truck's gas tank before you go on with your route. What is the quickest legal way to the gas station?
   a. west on Maple Street, north on 11th Avenue, and west on Oak Street to the entrance
   b. west on Maple Street, north on 9th Avenue, and west on Brown Street to the entrance
   c. east on Maple Street, north on 9th Avenue, and west on Brown Street to the entrance
   d. east on Maple Street, north on 10th Avenue, and west on Oak Street to the entrance

44. As you are making a scheduled pickup at the clinic, a student comes up to you on foot and tells you he is new in town and wants to go to the library. He knows it's very close, but can't remember the name of the street he should turn onto. You both walk around to the clinic door, and you advise him on the best route by telling him to
   a. walk to the corner of 10th Avenue and north one block to the library
   b. walk to the corner of Green Street and down Green Street to the library
   c. walk to the corner of Brown Street and down Brown Street to the library
   d. walk to the corner of 11th Avenue, and north one block to the library

45. The directions on an exam allow $2\frac{1}{2}$ hours to answer 50 questions. If you want to spend an equal amount of time on each of the 50 questions, about how much time should you allow for each one?

   a. 45 seconds
   b. $1\frac{1}{2}$ minutes
   c. 2 minutes
   d. 3 minutes

46. You've been assigned to pick up waste that is labeled hazardous. The rules for handling this hazardous material tell you to wear a respirator, goggles, and special gloves before moving these containers. You discover that you've forgotten to check out a respirator. What should you do?
   a. hold your breath while carrying the container to the truck
   b. tie a piece of cloth around your mouth and breath through it
   c. do not go near the material until you get a respirator
   d. throw a towel over the container and then carry it over to the truck

47. The department's policy of aggressively recruiting women drivers is <u>unique</u>. In this sentence, the word <u>unique</u> most nearly means
   a. rigorous
   b. admirable
   c. unparalleled
   d. remarkable

48. While collecting recyclables at 804 Olive Street, Sanitation Worker Johnston slips on an icy sidewalk and twists his right ankle. As he is trying to get up, a passerby, Ed Willard, stops his car and offers to help. Johnston is in pain and soon realizes that he cannot put weight on his ankle. Willard offers to take Johnston to the hospital and helps him into his car. When Johnston sees Willard's car phone, he asks if he can call his supervisor. Which of the following reports describes the situation most clearly and accurately?

  a. I fell on the ice at 804 Olive Street. I injured my ankle and may need medical treatment. I am phoning from the car of a man who stopped to help me.

  b. I am in Ed Willard's car, who helped me when I was collecting at 804 Olive Street. My right ankle might be a problem.

  c. I cannot put any weight on my right ankle where I fell when collecting some recyclables. I am waiting in Ed Willard's car.

  d. Ed Willard on Olive Street helped me as I was collecting, twisting an ankle, which may need the emergency room.

49. All trucks must carry four triangle-shaped reflectors and a first aid kit at all times. You are late to work one morning, so you hurry through your pre-trip inspection. You notice that your truck only has one reflector. What should you do?

  a. take three reflectors out of a nearby truck and put them back at the end of your shift

  b. run your route without the three reflectors— chances are you won't need them

  c. ask the maintenance supervisor for three more reflectors and put them in your truck

  d. run part of your route to make up the time you've lost, and then come back and pick up the three reflectors

50. You are running a new route today, and you have a helper with you. Your helper is signaling that it is safe for you to back the truck up. Even though the helper is signaling that the way is clear, you see something in your mirror that makes you think it isn't. What should you do?

  a. back up anyway; since the helper is outside the truck, he is probably right

  b. change places with the helper and have him back up the truck

  c. get out of the truck and check the situation out for yourself before backing

  d. call a supervisor and ask for a third opinion before backing

51. County Sanitation Department policy states that tires will be picked up by special collection on request of a resident. There is a $3.50 charge for each tire collected. Residents may also take tires to the county landfill, where all tires will be accepted for a fee of 8¢ per pound. Sanitation Worker Yates is making a regular collection at 19 Center Road where there are two tires next to the trash can. The resident, Mr. Harper, comes out of the building and insists that Yates take the tires. Yates explains the policy. Which explanation most clearly and accurately describes the department policy?

  a. If you want your tires collected, make a special request at the landfill. You will be charged $3.50 or 8¢ a pound.

  b. To have tires picked up, you must request a special collection. The charge is $3.50 per tire. You may also take tires to the landfill, where the charge is 8¢ per pound.

  c. We do not collect tires unless you pay a fee of $3.50 per tire. The other choice is to take your tires to the landfill and have them weighed.

  d. Since you have two tires you will be charged $7.00 each if you make a special request or if you take the tires to the landfill.

52. Sanitation Worker O'Rourke has just finished collecting at 639 Evans Road. He is stopped behind a small Toyota pickup truck that is parked in a no parking zone. As O'Rourke tries to pull his collection truck around the pickup, he accidentally hits the back of it and breaks the pickup's left taillight. O'Rourke phones in a report to his supervisor. Which of the following reports most clearly and accurately describes the incident?

   a. I broke a taillight on the truck. It was parked in a no parking zone at 639 Evans Road.

   b. As I was leaving 639 Evans Road, I hit the back of a Toyota pickup truck and broke one of its taillights.

   c. Because I was leaving 639 Evans Road in a no parking zone, I hit a Toyota which broke one of its lights.

   d. The Toyota was in a no parking zone and since I couldn't get around it, I hit it. This all took place at 936 Evans Road.

53. If it takes two workers 2 hours 40 minutes to complete a particular task, about how long will it take one worker to complete the same task alone?

   a. 1 hour 20 minutes

   b. 4 hours 40 minutes

   c. 5 hours

   d. 5 hours 20 minutes

54. You are emptying containers along a busy city sidewalk. As you lift one container you look down and find a baby wrapped in a towel inside the container. The baby starts to cry. What should you do?

   a. put the baby in the truck and drive it to the nearest hospital as quickly as possible

   b. call for police and medical help, then ask one of the store owners to wait with the baby while you continue on your route

   c. leave your helper behind to wait with the baby for the authorities to come, and then continue your route

   d. radio your dispatcher to send police and medical help to your location and wait for them to arrive

55. If a worker is given a salary increase of $1.25 per hour, what it the total amount of the salary increase for one 40-hour week?

   a. $49.20

   b. $50.00

   c. $50.25

   d. $51.75

56. Which of the items shown below could most easily be carried by one person?

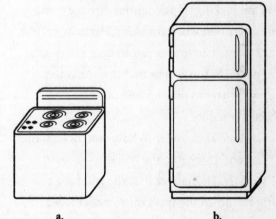

a.   b.

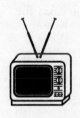
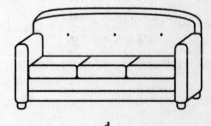

c.   d.

Answer question 57 based on the procedure below.

Safe backing is a major concern for sanitation workers. Before backing up a truck you should check the area as you drive into position, get out of the cab and check the area directly behind the truck before backing, and use both rear view and side mirrors constantly while the truck is moving.

57. Sanitation Worker Harridan is pulling into the yard after a long day at work. Other trucks are arriving also. Harridan drives her truck to her usual parking spot and positions the truck for backing. What should she do next?
   a. back slowly and carefully into the slot
   b. get out and check to make sure nothing is in the way before backing
   c. honk once and back quickly into the slot
   d. wait for the next truck to pull in so that driver can wave her on back

58. You are picking up residential garbage alone one afternoon when frail Mrs. Hernandez from 1212 Garza Circle asks you to take a large carton of trash. You realize that the box is too heavy for you to pick up on your own. What should you do?
   a. ask Mrs. Hernandez to help you pick up the box and carry it to the truck
   b. tell Mrs. Hernandez that she will have to break down the trash into smaller loads
   c. alternate picking up and scooting the box because that is your job
   d. ask a male neighbor to help you carry the box to the truck

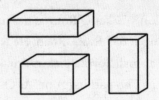

59. The fastest and easiest way to move the boxes shown above a short distance is

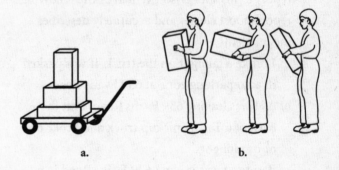

a.   b.

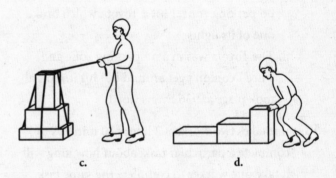

c.   d.

60. It's time for a lunch break and you pull up to the Spud Bud for lunch. Company policy states that, if you leave your truck unattended, you must place wooden blocks behind the wheels to prevent the truck from rolling. You know your truck has a good emergency brake, and you are picking up your food to go and won't be inside for long. What should you do?
   a. set the brake, run inside, and watch out the window while they fix your order
   b. put the blocks under the wheels of the truck before you go inside the restaurant

c. back up against the building so the truck won't hit anything if it does roll

d. parallel park the truck between two cars so it cannot roll

61. The most common injury suffered by sanitation workers is muscle strain. The best way to avoid pulling a muscle is to warm up your muscles, so your supervisor reminds you every morning to warm up before heading out on your route. What should you do?

a. drink a warm cup of coffee or tea before getting on the truck

b. loosen your muscles with warm-up exercises at the end of the day

c. loosen your muscles with warm-up exercises before starting your route

d. for the first few minutes of your route, turn the heater inside the truck to high

62. The city ordinance states that there is to be no open burning within the city limits. While Sanitation Worker Holt is collecting trash at 340 Phillips Street, she notices that a man across the street at 341 Phillips is burning trash and leaves in his yard. As she has been instructed to do, she reports the incident to the city's fire department. Which of the following reports describes the incident most clearly and accurately?

a. Someone is breaking the no burning law by burning leaves and trash on Phillips Street.

b. While I was collecting at 340 Phillips Street, I saw a pile of leaves and trash burning openly.

c. There is a man burning leaves and trash in his yard at 341 Phillips Street.

d. The house at 341 Phillips Street has been burning from the trash and leaves in the yard.

63. You are driving a front end loader that lifts dumpsters over the cab of the truck to empty them. You see that nearby construction crews have strung temporary power lines near a dumpster that you are scheduled to pick up this morning, and you do not believe you have enough room to lift it. What should you do?

a. have your helper assist you in emptying the dumpster out by hand

b. ask the construction crew to help you empty the dumpster out by hand, since they are the ones causing the problem

c. empty the dumpster with the truck—if any wires are knocked down, it is the construction crew's responsibility to put them back up

d. do not attempt to empty this dumpster and notify your supervisor of the problem

64. A street sign reads "Loading Zone 15 Minutes." If a truck pulls into this zone at 11:46 a.m., by what time must it leave?

a. 11:59 a.m.

b. 12:01 p.m.

c. 12:03 p.m.

d. 12:06 p.m.

65. You are unloading a dumpster when the lifting mechanism jams. You can't lower or raise the dumpster and it is hanging right above the cab of your truck. What should you do?

a. radio the dispatcher and ask for help to be sent out

b. drive the truck to the repair yard with the dumpster half-raised above the truck

c. try to shake the mechanism loose by backing up and stepping on the brakes quickly and firmly

d. climb up onto the dumpster and jump up and down on it to release the jam

66. A container, when empty, weighs 27 pounds. If this container is filled with a load of trash that weighs 108 pounds, what is the total weight of the container and its contents?
a. 81 pounds
b. 135 pounds
c. 145 pounds
d. 185 pounds

67. The documentation of Sanitation Worker Martinez's excellent driving record was <u>meticulous</u>. In this sentence, the word <u>meticulous</u> most nearly means
a. delicate
b. responsible
c. objective
d. painstaking

68. Which of the following figures is the figure shown above, turned in a different position?

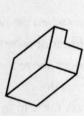
a.

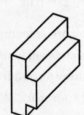
b.

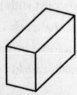
c.

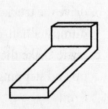
d.

69. While driving your route on Sandy Hill Way one day, you pass a group of neighborhood children, who appear to be 12 or 13 years old, rollerblading in the street close to the curb. After you finish your pickups, because of deep potholes in the street ahead, you realize that it would be more convenient and easier on your vehicle if you back down Sandy Hill Way, rather than continuing on around the block. What should you do?
a. ask one of the kids to keep the others safe as you back up the truck
b. back up slowly—the kids are old enough to get out of the way safely
c. drive around the block slowly, to minimize jolting of your vehicle
d. back up in the middle of the street as the kids are rollerblading close to the curb

70. An elevator sign reads "Maximum weight 600 pounds." Which of the following may ride the elevator?
a. three people: one weighing 198 pounds, one weighing 185 pounds, one weighing 200 pounds
b. one person weighing 142 pounds with a load weighing 500 pounds
c. one person weighing 165 pounds with a load weighing 503 pounds
d. three people: one weighing 210 pounds, one weighing 101 pounds, one weighing 298 pounds.

ANSWERS

1. **c.** Since Wallace has recognized that the signal light is probably hanging too low for his truck to fit under, he should change lanes and move around it.

2. **a.** Ammand is driving an unfamiliar vehicle, and if he's not sure it will fit under the overhang, he is required to get out and look before making the turn. Driving on the sidewalk is not permissible. Waiting for a dispatcher to call the building owner will take too long, as will waiting for his regular truck to be fixed.

3. **d.** This is the only clear and accurate report. Choice **a** doesn't report why Marshall will be late. Choice **b** doesn't say Marshall will be late for work. Choice **c** doesn't say what happened.

4. **d.** This is the only even number and therefore the only east-west route. The other choices are north-south routes.

5. **a.** Always get out and check if you don't know if your truck will fit in, under, or around any obstacle. You should never choose an option that puts you or anyone else at risk, so having your helper stand on top of the crate is not a good answer. And you wouldn't want a high-voltage power line to touch any part of your truck no matter how fast you are going. To wait for the power company to fix the problem will take too much time.

6. **a.** This is a two-step subtraction problem. First you must find out how many miles the truck has traveled since its last maintenance. To do this subtract 12,398 from 22,003. Then, take the answer, 9,605, and subtract it from 13,000 to find out how many more miles the truck can travel before it must have another maintenance: 3,395.

7. **b.** The answer is found in the third sentence. Choice **a** is incorrect because there is no mention

of plastic bags in the passage. Choices **c** and **d** are incorrect because it is the people in their homes—not the sanitation workers—who use the sharp objects and fail to mark the containers.

8. **a.** Notification must be made one hour before the shift begins—which would be 6:30. The other choices give incorrect times.

9. **d.** Taking the time to adjust one mirror might mean the difference between finishing your route safely and running into something. Your best choice is to fix the mirror and then back up.

10. **c.** This is the only accurate report. None of the other choices accurately state the exact nature of the problem or where the problem is located.

11. **b.** Something that is *intermittent* is periodic—i.e., it stops and starts at intervals.

12. **b.** The procedure for safe lifting states that Spagenberg should have both feet flat on the ground and should tip the container a little to see how heavy it is before picking it up.

13. **d.** To pick up this load, Graviel should follow the rules by facing the box and keeping both feet on the ground and both knees unlocked.

14. **c.** Choices **a** and **b** should be poured into the sewer system; choice **d** should be saved for a special collection.

15. **b.** Because the can is not empty, it should not be placed in the trash. It contains bug spray, which should be saved for a special collection.

16. **a.** Choices **b** and **d** should be dried out and placed in the trash; choice **c** should be saved for a special collection.

17. **a.** This is a simple subtraction problem. $5\frac{1}{2}$ minus 3 is $2\frac{1}{2}$.

18. **b.** This is the only clear and accurate statement. None of the other choices even indicate that Jarvis

was driving the truck. Choice **d** does not say where the accident took place.

19. d. No one likes to work in the rain, but the job does mean getting wet on some occasions. Since you have no idea when the rain will stop, it's up to you in this case to do your job now in a timely manner.

20. a. Safety First should be your battle cry. In this situation your helper's physical well-being is more important that any other consideration. Get medical attention for your helper. It's inappropriate to ask for assistance from someone who does not work for the department, and besides, lifting the sofa could injure that person.

21. a. Exams are only given on June 3, 6, 17, and 20, and the 17th is after the employee plans to start working, so **a** is the only possible choice.

22. d. June 24 is the fourth Tuesday of the month, and no exams are given.

23. c. You must subtract the reading at the beginning of the week from the reading at the end of the week. 21,053 minus 20,907 is 146.

24. c. This is the only clear and accurate report. Choice **a** does not say that Caruso was rescuing the kitten. Choice **b** sounds as though the boy made the scratch. Choice **d** is unclear.

25. b. Though the passage does not directly state that fatigue causes a person to become less alert, it does imply this in the fifth sentence.

26. d. The answer is found in the last sentence of the passage. Choices **a**, **b**, and **c** are not mentioned in the passage.

27. a. This is the only clear and accurate statement. Choice **b** implies that the building could explode. Choice **c** fails to give the exact location. Choice **d** doesn't mention that there is possibly an explosive in the dumpster.

28. c. In choice **a**, a right onto State does not lead to Washington. Choices **b** and **d** would mean traveling the wrong way on a one-way street.

29. b. Using the directional guide for the map, it is easy to see that northwest is the only possible answer.

30. b. In this situation you should not risk driving forward without direction from the helper. Although the helper's job usually entails directing you when you back up, it's unlikely that sanitation department rules would limit the job solely to that. Having the helper run behind the truck won't help because you are working with equipment on the front end. The other choices aren't safe.

31. d. This is the only clear and accurate account of what happened. Choice **a** implies that Lopez was accused of theft. Choice **b** gives an incorrect location. Choice **c** is unclear and inaccurate.

32. b. This is a two-step problem. First, add the three numbers, then divide the sum by 3 to find the average. 21 plus 18 plus 24 is 63, and 63 divided by 3 is 21.

33. a. Ron has not met the requirements because the application cannot be received at the department by March 1.

34. a. Something that is *tentative* is uncertain or provisional.

35. b. According to the chart, on Wednesday each of the trucks dumped five loads.

36. d. According to the chart, on Friday M-459 dumped six loads. Choices **a** and **c** are each four loads; choice **b** is five loads.

37. d. Carrying the load from west to east across the courtyard is the shortest distance to the back of the truck.

38. c. To be *incredulous* is to be skeptical or disbelieving.

39. a. According to the map, the other routes are impossible or illegal.

40. c. Brown Street and Park Street are the two streets that run north and south of the park.

41. a. According to the map, the other routes are impossible or illegal.

42. b. According to the map, choices **c** and **d** are impossible; choice **a** is circuitous.

43. d. Choices **a** and **b** take you the wrong way on Maple Street. Choice **c** will not get you to the entrance of the gas station.

44. d. According to the map, the other routes will not get the student to the library.

45. d. First convert the $2\frac{1}{2}$ hours to minutes. Then divide the answer by 50. 2 hours 30 minutes is 150 minutes. 150 divided by 50 is 3.

46. c. Get a respirator from the proper source. None of the other options is safe and all violate the rules.

47. c. If something is *unique*, it is one of a kind or unparalleled.

48. a. This is the only clear and accurate statement. Choices **b** and **c** do not clearly say what the injury was. Choice **d** implies that Ed Willard may have been injured.

49. c. It's your responsibility to make sure your truck is properly equipped. Your best choice is to take enough time to correctly handle this problem by getting the reflectors from the right source.

50. c. Your helper's name won't be entered in the "at fault" section of an accident report if you back into something—but your name will be! It's always best to check for yourself if you have any doubts.

51. b. This is the only clear and accurate statement of the policy. Choice **a** gives incorrect information. Choice **c** leaves out important information. Choice **d** states the policy incorrectly.

52. b. This is the only clear and accurate report. Choice **a** is unclear and doesn't say which truck was hit. Choice **c** is inaccurate. Choice **d** gives an incorrect address.

53. d. It will take one worker about twice as long. First add the hours and minutes. Four hours 80 minutes is equal to 5 hours 20 minutes.

54. d. The baby is your responsibility until help arrives. Since the child is crying, you can be sure that it is breathing, which would be your most immediate concern. Because you cannot be sure of the child's condition otherwise, it's best to not touch it until help reaches you.

55. b. This is a multiplication problem. $1.25 times 40 is $50.00.

56. c. The television is small and light enough for one person to carry. Choices **a** and **b** would most likely require two or more persons to move. Choice **d** might be pushed by one person, but the television is still the one that could *most easily* be moved.

57. b. The rule says the driver should get out of the cab and check behind the truck before backing.

58. b. Given the options that were listed here, it's best for you to tell Ms. Hernandez to break down the trash into smaller loads. You should never pick up an object that is too heavy—putting yourself at risk of injury is not part of your job. Asking a person who does not work for the sanitation department to help would be inappropriate and might put that person at risk of injury.

59. a. The fastest and easiest way is to move all the boxes together with a dolly. The other choices would either take longer or be more difficult.

60. b. Always follow department policy. Even if it seems unlikely, it's possible your truck could roll while you are inside the restaurant. A moment's laziness could very well endanger the lives of others or at the very least cost you your job. Depending on the building or other cars to stop the truck would not show good judgment.

61. c. Loosening your muscles *before* you start your shift will help you avoid muscle strain. Drinking a hot beverage may make your insides warm, but won't do much for your muscles—nor will the truck's heater be of much help.

62. c. This is the only clear and accurate report. Choice **a** does not give the exact address. Choice **b** implies that the burning is at 340 Phillips. Choice **d** implies that a house is on fire.

63. d. Skip this dumpster and let your supervisor untangle the situation. You should not unload dumpsters by hand or ask anyone else to do so, and emptying a dumpster is not worth the risk of electrocution.

64. b. If it is 11:46 a.m., in 14 minutes it will be noon. In 15 minutes, then, it will be 12:01.

65. a. Driving the truck in this condition is not safe, nor is any attempt to climb on top of the dumpster. Your best bet is to ask for help.

66. b. This is a simple addition problem. 108 plus 27 is 135.

67. d. To be *meticulous* is to be extremely careful and precise, or painstaking.

68. a. If you look carefully at choices **b**, **c**, and **d**, you will see that the shapes are not the same.

69. c. Backing up is one of the most dangerous maneuvers you can perform in any vehicle, and when there are children nearby it is rarely a good idea! Going around the block is the safest option for you in this situation. If you go slowly you will not damage your vehicle.

70. a. By rounding off the numbers, it is easy to see that choice **a** is less than 600 pounds and choices **b**, **c**, and **d** are all over 600 pounds.

SCORING

In order to score your exam, review the suggestions at the end of the second exam, Chapter 11.

If you didn't score as well as you would like on this third exam, be sure to try to analyze the reasons why. Ask yourself the following questions: Did I run out of time before I could answer all the questions? Did I go back and change my answers from right to wrong? Did I get flustered and sit staring at a hard question for what seemed like hours? If you had any of these problems, be sure to go over the test-taking strategies in Chapter 4 again to learn how to avoid them.

Finally, examine again how you did on each kind of question on the test in order to spot where your strengths and weaknesses lie. That way you'll know which areas require special effort in the time you have left before the exam. The table on this page identifies which questions on the third practice exam fall into which categories and lets you know which chapters to review if you had trouble with a particular type.

Keep in mind that self-confidence is the key, and that in using this book, you're making yourself better prepared than many of the other people taking the exam with you. Having taken practice exams, analyzed where your strengths and weaknesses lie, and learned how to approach the various kinds of questions on the test, you can go into the test with confidence.

SANITATION WORKER PRACTICE EXAM 3

Question Type	Question Numbers	Chapter
Reading	4, 7, 8, 14–16, 21, 22, 25, 26, 33, 35, 36	6, "Reading Comprehension"
Clarity	3, 10, 18, 24, 27, 31, 48, 51, 52, 62	7, "Verbal Expression"
Vocabulary	11, 34, 38, 47, 67	7, "Verbal Expression"
Map reading	28, 29, 39–44	8, "Map-Reading and Spatial Relations"
Spatial relations	37, 56, 59, 68	8, "Map-Reading and Spatial Relations"
Judgment and application of procedure	1, 2, 5, 9, 12, 13, 19, 20, 30, 46, 49, 50, 54, 57, 58, 60, 61, 63, 65, 69	9, "Good Judgment and Common Sense"
Math	6, 17, 23, 32, 45, 53, 55, 64, 66, 70	10, "Mathematics"

C·H·A·P·T·E·R

THE PHYSICAL TEST

13

CHAPTER SUMMARY

Not all hiring agencies require sanitation workers to pass a physical test as part of the hiring process. For those that do, this chapter reviews the demanding physical test that applicants have to take and pass to become a Sanitation Worker in New York City. It offers a complete rundown of the five events that make up the test plus helpful tips on preparing for this type of test.

A lthough sanitation work may seem simple on the surface, it demands a lot physically: balance, coordination, and stamina. You'll have to lug heavy cans or bags of garbage around, through, or over any number of obstacles, including parked cars and snowbanks. Efficiency is also crucial here: when you're on the job, you'll be assigned a collection route, and your team will be expected to complete the route in a certain amount of time. All of these job factors demand your top physical performance on a day to day basis.

The physical test is a set of what are called "job simulation tasks" because they mirror the day to day duties of sanitation workers. The test evaluates your physical capabilities that relate directly to the job: lifting, carrying, going around obstacles, and dragging. Because you'll have to perform all the tasks exactly as described by your test examiner, the test also determines your ability to follow directions. Your efficiency also factors into your success on the test: three of the events are timed. This means that you'll have to complete the tasks in these events within a certain amount of time.

PERFORMANCE COUNTS

To take the physical test, you first must score 70 percent or better on the Sanitation Worker written exam. The New York City Department of Citywide Administrative Services (DCAS), formerly the New York City Department of Personnel, creates an eligibility list of candidates who pass the written exam and then randomly selects a certain number of people from this list to take the physical test. The DCAS handles physical testing this way due to the volume of applicants for the job: the last time the exam was held, in 1990, 100,000 people took the written test. At that time, about 15,000 people were selected to participate in the physical test. The DCAS reports that in 1997, up to 30,000 people may be chosen.

A candidate's performance on the physical test has a direct impact on the Department of Sanitation's hiring considerations. The physical test determines your rank on the final eligibility list from which candidates are selected to fill sanitation worker positions. The message is simple: the higher your score on the physical test, the better your chances are of being hired.

Each event in the test counts one point, which means that the highest score you can get is five. You've only got one shot at passing this test!

TEST DAY

When you arrive at the test site (the DCAS will provide you with complete information on the address, date, and time of the physical test), you'll present a $10 testing fee (this is payable by money order only, made out to the New York City Department of Citywide Administrative Services). This fee is separate from the fee you submit to take the written exam.

For the physical test, it's best to wear loose-fitting work clothes for freedom of movement and shoes with a gripping sole. Athletic shoes are fine, but you may choose to wear lace-up boots for the additional ankle support you may need for carrying heavy items. Because this test requires a substantial amount of lifting, a weightlifter-style waist belt adds reinforcement to your lower back and can protect it from injury. You'll be provided with a set of gloves to use during the test.

THE PHYSICAL TEST

The accompanying chart shows the five events that make up the physical test.

YOUR PHYSICAL TEST
Event
1: Ladder Climb
2: Basket Retrieval
3: Emptying Street Corner Baskets
4: Drag or Carry Garbage Through Obstacles
5: Drag or Carry Garbage and Mattress to Sanitation Truck

The following pages describe in detail the five events of the physical test as it was given in 1990. As this book goes to press in November of 1996, it is expected that the 1997 physical test will remain essentially the same. Candidates should be able to perform tasks similar to the ones described below, as they are a lot like the job of a sanitation worker.

Event One: Ladder Climb

For the first event, you'll climb and descend a permanently secured 10-foot ladder. First you stand at a starting line about two feet from the ladder. At the examiner's signal, you climb up to a ladder rung from which you can see two hand-holds on a platform at the top of the ladder. After getting yourself up onto the platform, you put your hands into the hand-holds, go back to the ladder and descend the ladder to the floor. In order to qualify in this event, you must face the ladder both going up and down, and put at least one foot on each rung while you are climbing and descending. In other words, you can't skip rungs or jump down from the ladder. This event assesses your coordination and ability to follow directions.

Practice: Find an extension ladder and place it against a wall. While wearing work boots and gloves, practice going up and down the ladder in the way you'll be required to in the test. Find the most comfortable way to ascend and descend the ladder, either by putting just one foot at a time on a rung as you climb, or by placing one foot and then the other on the same rung before stepping up to the next one.

Event Two: Basket Retrieval

This event involves dragging an empty street-corner basket weighing 30 pounds over to a garbage truck and then back to the starting position. This test measures your upper body, leg, and hand-grip strength.

You'll start by standing about two feet away from the basket. At the examiner's signal, you drag the empty basket a distance of eight feet and step over a line on the floor with at least one foot. You'll lift the basket, place it on its side into a simulated sanitation truck, and remove both hands from the basket. You then take the basket out of the truck and drag it back to the starting position.

Practice: Create a space that can serve as a simulated sanitation truck, such as a row of folding chairs or an old desk, and measure a distance of eight feet between the "truck" and a starting position. Place a bag containing 30 pounds of sand into a large trash can and, while wearing gloves, drag the garbage can from the starting position to the truck, put it into and take it out of the truck, and return it to the starting position. Your goal is to accomplish this task as smoothly as possible.

Event Three: Empty Street Corner Baskets

Event Three, which is timed, consists of two sets of tasks that are performed consecutively. You must complete this event within 3.5 minutes.

The first set of tasks involves emptying five street-corner baskets filled with "garbage." For the second set of tasks, you'll carry filled baskets to a truck by going around an obstacle, then empty the baskets, and return them to the starting position.

For the first part of this event, the examiner will give you a signal and begin timing you. You'll drag the first filled street basket eight feet to a sanitation truck. This basket contains a bag that weighs three pounds (remember, the basket itself weighs 30 pounds). You step over a line on the floor with at least one foot, lift the basket, empty its contents into the truck, and then return the empty basket to the starting position. After you have returned the first basket, you perform the same task with a second, third, and fourth basket, each filled with a bag that weighs five, 15, and 13 pounds, respectively. The fifth basket, which you must also take to the truck, contains a 35-pound bag that you must lift *directly from* the basket and place in the truck (note that baskets 1-4 may be lifted and dumped into the truck). You may leave the fifth basket upright or place it on its side before removing the bag. You then take the basket back to the starting position.

After you return the fifth basket to the starting position, you proceed immediately to the next half of Event Three. This second set of tasks is similar to the first, except you'll have to maneuver around an obstacle to get the baskets to and from the truck.

You'll drag (one at a time) five filled baskets to a sanitation truck by following a marked route around an obstacle, step over a line on the floor with at least one foot, lift the basket, and empty its contents into the truck. Following the marked route, you return it to the starting position. The first four baskets contain bags that weigh three, five, 13, and 25 pounds, respectively. The fifth basket, filled with a 33-pound bag, is handled like the fifth basket in the first set of tasks. You can't lift the basket to empty it. Instead, you must remove the bag directly from the basket and place the bag in the truck. You may leave the basket upright or lay it on its side before removing the bag. The examiner will stop the clock when you have returned the fifth basket to the starting position.

After you complete Event Three, you are directed to an area where you take a two-minute rest period. When the rest period is over, you begin Event Four.

Practice: The point to this practice exercise is to build up your lifting capability, endurance, and your arm, leg, upper body, and grip strength.

Fill pillowcases or garbage bags with books or other heavy items and put the pillowcases or bags into five large trash cans.

Using the simulated sanitation truck again, practice taking increasingly heavy cans to the truck while wearing gloves. Next, set a chair or some other obstacle in the path from the starting position to the truck and carry the bags to the truck by going around the obstacle. Have a friend use a stop watch to time you, and work to get your time as low as possible.

Another good practice exercise that will strengthen your leg muscles is to run up flights of stairs with a filled knapsack on your back. This will also increase your endurance, which is crucial for this event.

Event Four: Drag or Carry Garbage Through Obstacles

Event Four consists of five tasks that require you to drag or carry six to eight items of garbage through, around, between, and over obstacles. You'll be timed in this event, and you'll have to complete all the tasks within five minutes.

Below is a chart that indicates the number of items and their weights for tasks one through five.

For the first task, you begin in the rest area where you had your two-minute rest period. At the examiner's signal, the clock is started. You drag or carry eight items of garbage to a simulated sanitation truck by going through an opening between two wooden boxes. You step over a line on the floor with at least one foot, and place the garbage into the truck. Three of these items weigh eight pounds, three weigh 15 pounds, and the other two weigh 25 and 45 pounds. You aren't expected to carry or drag all eight pieces at one time, but you may take more than one item per trip to the truck. You may not rest the garbage on the wooden boxes on the way to the truck.

The second task requires you carry or drag eight pieces of garbage to the truck by going over an obstacle

EVENT #4: ITEM QUANTITY & WEIGHTS		
Task	**Number of Items**	**Weights**
1	8	8, 8, 8, 15, 15, 15, 25, 45
2	8	8, 8, 15, 15, 15, 15, 25, 45
3	8	8, 8, 8, 15, 25, 25, 25, 35
4	6	8, 15, 15, 15, 25, 65
5	7	8, 15, 15, 15, 25, 35, 35

simulating a snow bank. You'll step over a line on the floor with at least one foot and put the items in the truck. Two of these items weigh eight pounds, four weigh 15 pounds, and the other two weigh 25 and 45 pounds.

For task number three, you'll carry or drag eight items of garbage to the truck by going around a wooden box. As in the prior tasks, you step over a line on the floor with one foot and place the items into the truck. Three of these items weigh eight pounds, one weighs 15 pounds, three weigh 25 pounds, and the last item weighs 35 pounds.

The fourth task involves carrying or dragging six items of garbage (weighing 8, 15, 15, 15, 25, and 65 pounds) between two wooden boxes, step over a line on the floor with at least one foot, and place the garbage in the truck.

The final task in Event Four requires you to carry or drag seven pieces of garbage (weighing 8, 15, 15, 15, 25, 35, and 35 pounds) over a railroad tie, step over a line on the floor with at least one foot, and place the items in the truck. The examiner will stop the clock when you have placed the last item of garbage in the truck. You are then directed to the rest area where you take a two-minute rest period.

Practice: The idea behind this event is to test your agility, stamina, and strength. To practice for it, set up an obstacle course for yourself, made up of objects you can walk through, step over, and go around. (Chairs, tables, pillows, or boxes make great obstacles.) Try tak-ing armloads of heavy objects to your simulated sanitation truck by going through the obstacle course.

One good way to build stamina (as well as balance and coordination) is to march up and down stairs carrying armloads of books, or even a small child!

Event Five: Drag or Carry Garbage and Mattress to a Sanitation Truck

To pass this event, you must carry or drag five sets of garbage items to a simulated sanitation truck, step over a line on the floor with at least one foot, and place the items in the truck. You'll also have to drag a full-size mattress a distance of eight feet to pass this event. The challenge of this event is the quantity and weight of the items you take to the truck. This is a timed event that you must complete within 6.5 minutes.

Below is a chart that indicates the number of items and their weights for tasks one through five (the sixth task, again, is the mattress drag).

The examiner will give you a signal and start the clock. You may carry or drag as many items as you wish at one time. You aren't expected to take all of them at once. After you place the last item into the truck, you proceed to the sixth task, in which you drag a mattress eight feet from the starting position, across a line drawn on the floor. The examiner will stop the clock when the mattress is completely across the line. When you have finished the test, you return the gloves and take a rest period before leaving the testing site.

EVENT #5: ITEM QUANTITY & WEIGHTS

Task	Number of Items	Weights
1	11	8, 8, 8, 8, 8, 8, 15, 15, 15, 25, 25
2	6	15, 15, 15, 25, 25, 45
3	7	8, 15, 15, 15, 25, 35, 55
4	7	8, 8, 15, 15, 25, 35, 35
5	6	8, 15, 15, 15, 25, 65

Practice: Because this event is similar to Event Four, you can use the practice exercise described under the fourth event to prepare for it. To practice for the mattress drag, if you don't have a mattress handy, try loading up a sheet with books and practice dragging it. The mattress drag tests your leg and grip strength.

Preparing for the physical test is crucial. If you begin a regular exercise program, stop smoking and reduce excessive alcohol intake, and use the practice exercises described in this chapter, you should be on your way to succeeding not only in the test, but in your career as a sanitation worker.

<u>NOTES</u>

NOTES

NOTES

NOTES

NOTES

<u>NOTES</u>

<u>NOTES</u>

NOTES

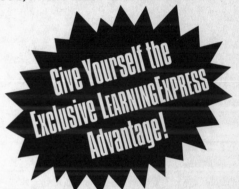

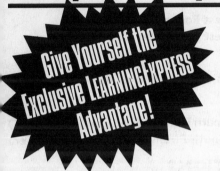